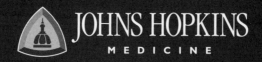
JOHNS HOPKINS
MEDICINE

Patients' Guide to
Breast Cancer

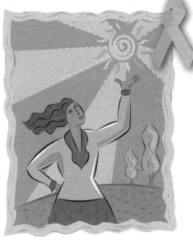

Lillie D. Shockney, RN, BS, MAS

*University Distinguished Service Assistant Professor of Breast Cancer; Administrative
Director of Breast Center; Assistant Professor, Department of Surgery; Assistant Professor,
Department of Obstetrics and Gynecology, Johns Hopkins School of Medicine
Assistant Professor, Johns Hopkins School of Nursing*

Series Editors

Lillie D. Shockney

Gary R. Shapiro, MD

Chairman, Department of Oncology

gy
nter
y Program
r at Johns Hopkins

D1004646

JONES AND BARTLETT PUBLISHERS
Sudbury, Massachusetts
BOSTON   TORONTO   LONDON   SINGAPORE

World Headquarters

Jones and Bartlett Publishers
40 Tall Pine Drive
Sudbury, MA 01776
978-443-5000
info@jbpub.com
www.jbpub.com

Jones and Bartlett Publishers
Canada
6339 Ormindale Way
Mississauga, Ontario L5V 1J2
Canada

Jones and Bartlett Publishers
International
Barb House, Barb Mews
London W6 7PA
United Kingdom

Jones and Bartlett's books and products are available through most bookstores and online booksellers. To contact Jones and Bartlett Publishers directly, call 800-832-0034, fax 978-443-8000, or visit our website www.jbpub.com.

Substantial discounts on bulk quantities of Jones and Bartlett's publications are available to corporations, professional associations, and other qualified organizations. For details and specific discount information, contact the special sales department at Jones and Bartlett via the above contact information or send an email to specialsales@jbpub.com.

The authors, editor, and publisher have made every effort to provide accurate information. However, they are not responsible for errors, omissions, or for any outcomes related to the use of the contents of this book and take no responsibility for the use of the products and procedures described. Treatments and side effects described in this book may not be applicable to all people; likewise, some people may require a dose or experience a side effect that is not described herein. Drugs and medical devices are discussed that may have limited availability controlled by the Food and Drug Administration (FDA) for use only in a research study or clinical trial. Research, clinical practice, and government regulations often change the accepted standard in this field. When consideration is being given to use of any drug in the clinical setting, the healthcare provider or reader is responsible for determining FDA status of the drug, reading the package insert, and reviewing prescribing information for the most up-to-date recommendations on dose, precautions, and contraindications, and determining the appropriate usage for the product. This is especially important in the case of drugs that are new or seldom used.

Production Credits
Executive Publisher: Christopher Davis
Senior Editorial Assistant: Jessica Acox
Production Director: Amy Rose
Production Assistant: Laura Almozara
Marketing Manager: Ilana Goddess
V.P., Manufacturing and Inventory Control: Therese Connell
Cover Design: Kristin E. Parker
Cover Image: © ImageZoo/age fotostock
Printing and Binding: Malloy, Inc.
Cover Printing: Malloy, Inc.

Library of Congress Cataloging-in-Publication Data

Shockney, Lillie, 1953–
    Johns Hopkins patients' guide to breast cancer / Lillie Shockney.
        p. cm.
    Includes index.
    ISBN-13: 978-0-7637-7426-4
    ISBN-10: 0-7637-7426-X
    1. Breast—Cancer—Popular works. I. Title. II. Title: Guide to breast cancer.
    RC280.B8S49516 2010
    616.99'449—dc22
                                                                                    2009007715

6048

Printed in the United States of America
13 12 11 10 09   10 9 8 7 6 5 4 3 2 1

Contents

Preface

Receiving a diagnosis of breast cancer is overwhelming. Trying to determine your next steps following the diagnosis can be equally paralyzing. Rather than entering an environment that is totally foreign to you, consider learning some information in advance.

With more than 250,000 individuals diagnosed with breast cancer in the United States in 2008, you are certainly not alone. Many have come before you, and still more will come after you. Empowering yourself with information is key to making informed decisions, participating in treatment choices presented to you by your oncology team, and gaining confidence that you are on the right track.

This book is part of a series of Johns Hopkins Cancer Patient Guides designed to educate newly-diagnosed patients about their cancer diagnosis and the treatment that may lie ahead. The information provided will guide patients and their support teams of family and friends from the time cancer is confirmed to the completion of treatment.

Don't feel the need to read the entire book at once. It is intended for you to read at your leisure and when you feel ready for additional information. Resource information, including access to Johns Hopkins oncology specialists, is also contained within these pages.

Until there is a cure and there are effective ways to prevent this disease, the medical team of the Johns Hopkins Breast Center will continue to support patients who hear the words "you have breast cancer."

Lillie D. Shockney, RN, BS, MAS
Seventeen-Year Breast Cancer Survivor
Distinguished Service Assistant Professor of Breast Cancer,
Johns Hopkins Avon Foundation Breast Center

DEDICATION

This book is dedicated to all newly-diagnosed breast cancer patients and their families. I hope the information contained within these pages empowers you so that you feel confident in the treatment plan that lies ahead. This life-altering journey is a profound experience for you and those who love you. I hope to see you in the future, at a breast cancer walk or other event celebrating your survivorship.

Lillie D. Shockney

INTRODUCTION

How to Use This Book to Your Benefit

You will receive a great deal of information from your healthcare team. You will also probably seek out some information on the Internet or in bookstores. No doubt friends and family members, meaning well, will offer you advice on what to do and when to do it, and will try to steer you in certain directions. Relax. Yes, you have heard words you wish you had never heard said about you, that you have breast cancer. Despite that shocking phrase, you have time to make good decisions and to empower yourself with accurate information so that you can participate in the decision making about your care and treatment.

This book is designed to be a "how-to" guide that will take you through the maze of treatment options and sometimes complicated schedules, and will help you put together a plan of action so that you become a breast cancer survivor. Eighty-five percent of women diagnosed today will be survivors of this disease. Your goal is to join that majority.

This book is broken down into chapters and includes an index as well as credible resources listed for your further review and education. By empowering yourself with understandable information, we hope you will be comfortable participating in the decision making about your treatment.

With the exception of only a few types of rare breast cancers, you don't need to rush into treatment immediately. You have time on your side to plan things well and confidently.

Let's begin now with understanding what has happened and what the steps are to get you well again.

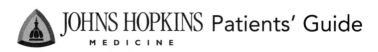

CHAPTER 1

JOHNS HOPKINS Patients' Guide
MEDICINE

First Steps—
I've Been Diagnosed
with Breast Cancer

You've recently had a breast biopsy or been told by a radiologist that the mass in your breast definitely looks like breast cancer. No doubt you are in shock having heard those words. Some women think such things as: "I don't have a family history of cancer, so how is this possible?"; "I don't have any risk factors, so how did I get it?"; and "I get my mammogram every year, so why do I have breast cancer?"

Let's begin by answering these common questions.

Family History: Only 12 percent of women diagnosed with breast cancer have a family history of the disease, meaning that 88 percent of women diagnosed with breast cancer have no breast cancer family history. Sometimes, however, patients get confused and assume that cancer of any kind in the family is the same as breast cancer history in the family. It is not. According to the American Cancer Society, one in three people in the United States will develop some type of cancer in their lifetime. Though most of these do not have a genetic link, there are certain cancers that do. If breast, ovarian, melanoma, or pancreatic cancers run in your family, you may want to discuss your risk of cancer with a genetics counselor. By and large, however, most women diagnosed with breast cancer have no familial history that predisposes them to getting this disease.

Risk Factors: Seventy percent of women diagnosed with breast cancer have no known risk factors. This means that there are some risk factors that medical experts simply don't know exist. Trying to guess them will exhaust you; it exhausts the researchers who are working hard to try to discover them on the behalf of all women.

Mammograms: Mammograms are not designed to prevent someone from getting breast cancer. Though their purpose is to identify breast cancer at the earliest moment it can be seen on an X-ray image, not every single cancer will be found on a mammogram. No X-ray or breast imaging technique is 100 percent perfect at detection. Mammography may not detect small tumors in women with dense breast tissue, and even if you have been getting regular mammograms, your tumor may not have been detected until it was relatively large. Still, mammography remains the gold standard for early detection. Smart women who get annual mammograms beginning at age 40 live longer than those who get them sporadically throughout their lives.

SELECTING YOUR ONCOLOGY TEAM AND BREAST CENTER

You want to be in the hands of experts. This isn't a simple gallbladder problem or hernia repair; this is cancer. Don't rely on self-promoting advertisements on television as a way to select a facility and doctor. Seek out an accredited (e.g., American College of Surgeons or National Cancer Institute) cancer center with a breast cancer program. Such a facility will have breast surgical oncologists (who are different from general surgeons who do some breast surgery as well as some hernia repairs and appendectomies), breast medical oncologists, breast radiation oncologists, breast pathologists, breast imaging radiologists, genetics counselors, oncology nurses, and psychosocial support staff for breast cancer patients. This group is highly specialized. Studies have confirmed that having your treatment done by breast cancer specialists provides you with a higher probability of survival than having it done by generalists. Ask your surgeon questions.

- How many breast cancer surgeries do you do a year?

- What is your breast conservation rate?

- What other types of surgeries do you do, and therefore how much of your time is spent doing breast cancer treatment? (You don't want a jack-of-all-trades and master of none.)

- Are you board certified in surgery?

- Do you specialize in cancer surgery as a surgical oncologist?

- How long have you been in practice? (This helps confirm the surgeon has the appropriate skills and training you may need.)

- Do you regularly attend breast cancer tumor boards to present cases for team discussion?

- Do you work with a multidisciplinary team of oncologists who also specialize in breast cancer so continuity of care can be maintained?

- What is your philosophy on educating patients about their treatment options?

- How many sentinel node biopsies have you performed?

- Do you have photographs of patients you have operated on so I can see mastectomy incisions, a mastectomy with reconstruction, and a lumpectomy? (See "Breast Cancer—Making the Right Choices for You" at http://www.hopkinsbreastcenter.org. This online document will provide you with more details about selecting the specialists you will need to help you in your fight against breast cancer.)

These are all questions you have the right to have answered before deciding that this doctor will be your breast surgical oncologist. If he or she hesitates about answering any question, consider that a sign that this person may not be the doctor you want to attempt to bond with and take the lead in helping you fight your breast cancer.

It's not unusual for a patient to get a second opinion after an initial consultation, particularly if she has initially gone to a smaller facility where breast oncology specialists may not be available.

LEARNING ABOUT YOUR DISEASE BEFORE THE FIRST VISIT

Here is some information that you should know at the outset:

- More than 80 percent of women are good candidates for breast-conserving surgery (lumpectomy) and don't have to lose their breast to this disease.
- Research studies show that women who seek emotional support during and after treatment have higher survival rates than those who decline to do so.
- Generally, the earlier you are diagnosed, the less treatment you will need to beat this disease.
- The side effects from adjuvant treatment (chemotherapy and radiation) can now be minimized with the use of drugs available for that purpose.
- Many women report that their lives are more fulfilled after a diagnosis of breast cancer than they were before.
- The majority of women work and continue their activities of daily living during treatment.

GATHERING RECORDS: BIOPSY, RADIOLOGY STUDIES, OTHER TESTS

As soon as you hear those words, "you have breast cancer," request a copy of the mammogram report and pathology's biopsy summary report. Be sure to obtain copies of all your medical records, and request copies as you continue along this journey so that you maintain your own portfolio of your care and treatment and test results. Begin with mammogram reports for the last 3 years, your current mammogram report, breast biopsy report, pathology report, and any other imaging done since you were diagnosed. This could be an ultrasound, a CAT scan, a breast MRI, or spot films in mammography. No matter who sees you—your surgeon, medical oncologist, or radiation oncologist—they will want to review these. They also need to see the actual films or images taken, so find out from the facility where the imaging was done and how to go about picking them up so you can bring them with you to your first consultation visit. Do the same with your pathology slides from your biopsy.

You might think, "Why do I need to get these things if my doctors have the reports?" An accredited cancer center is required to review the images and most specifically the pathology slides to verify their accuracy. There are situations in which review by a specialist in breast pathology reveals an error was made and that instead of invasive breast cancer, the patient has noninvasive disease. Of course, the opposite situation is also possible, and the breast pathologist may change the diagnosis from "benign" or noninvasive to invasive breast cancer. Accuracy is key for pathology. Your treatment plan at every step is based on this information being correct.

LEARNING THE PATHOLOGY FINDINGS AND CLINICAL DETAILS OF YOUR BREAST CANCER

Initially, all the information on your medical reports and that from your doctor may sound like Greek to you. By the end of your treatment, however, you will be quoting this information yourself with confidence and knowledge. Some women say they think they can write their own encyclopedia on this disease when they finish their treatment—and it's probably true.

Before you visit your doctor, let's further jump-start your knowledge base a bit by reviewing the pathology findings from your breast biopsy. The majority of biopsies are done as core biopsies and provide a tiny window into the big picture that is soon to be uncovered. This piece of tissue provides information about the type of breast cancer you have and a few specifics about its characteristics. It isn't intended to tell much more than this. The surgery that will be performed will answer the other important prognostic questions. So, until then, it can be premature to ask the doctor too much about your prognosis, the exact stage of the disease (beyond what is called clinical staging; not pathology staging), and precisely what the details of your treatment will be. Along with information from your breast imaging studies, the biopsy information provides your doctors with what is needed to determine your surgical treatment recommendations.

There are two primary types of invasive breast cancer. You can research others that are diagnosed less frequently on websites like http://www.breastcancer.org or http://www.hopkinsbreastcenter.org, but for our purposes for now, let's begin with the major categories: invasive/infiltrating ductal carcinoma and invasive/infiltrating lobular carcinoma. Eighty-five percent of invasive cancers in breast cancer are ductal, and 12 percent are lobular.

"Ductal" means that the disease started in the ducts of the breast and then spread into the nearby fatty tissue of the breast. "Lobular" means that the disease started in the lobules of the breast. There are situations in which the pathology report will label the cells as mammary carcinoma. In this case, there is a mixture of ductal and lobular cancer cells together. "Invasive," however, does not always mean that the cancer has spread outside of the breast. Checking the lymph nodes (known as sentinel node biopsy) and reviewing the other prognostic factors during surgery help to determine the risk of this having happened.

The treatment of invasive breast cancers is the same, no matter where the cancer "started"—duct or lobule. The size of ductal carcinomas usually is fairly easy to estimate on a mammogram or ultrasound. Lobular carcinomas, however, can be a little trickier and can be smaller or larger than they appear on an X-ray image. Breast MRI sometimes is helpful to clarify a measurement, but the only way to accurately determine the tumor's size is for the pathologist to measure it in the tissue that the surgeon removes.

There is also a type of breast cancer called noninvasive carcinoma. This is breast cancer at the earliest stage at which it can be found. It is known as ductal carcinoma in situ (DCIS). The ductal cancer cells are limited to the lining of the duct, remaining at their original site, and have not yet become invasive. This type of cancer usually cannot be felt as a lump and can be seen only on a mammogram, which is why women are encouraged to get annual mammograms—to find cancer at this stage (Stage 0).

A point of confusion is with the term lobular carcinoma in situ (LCIS). Although the word carcinoma is used, it doesn't actually refer to cancer, but rather to a marker for predicting risk of developing breast cancer in the future. Women with this type of cell found on biopsy are usually referred to a high-risk specialist for further evaluation and should not be told they have cancer.

A rarer form of breast cancer is inflammatory breast cancer. The cancer cells are actually in the skin of the breast. The pathology report usually will say that there are dermal lymphatic cells among the cancer cells taken from a biopsy of the breast skin. This is known to be a more aggressive form of breast cancer and presents quite differently on clinical examination, usually with the presence of a rash on the breast and a normal mammogram.

The grade of the cells may also be recorded as part of the pathology report. Grades are 1, 2, or 3.

   1 = Slow growing and may be referred to as well-differentiated cells

   2 = Average growing and may be called moderately-differentiated cells

   3 = Rapidly growing and may be termed poorly-differentiated cells

Don't be surprised if your report says grade 3; some are. This doesn't mean cells are growing extraordinarily fast and you have an emergency on your hands. The term is used relatively.

9

There are additional tests that are more commonly done on the cancer specimen that is removed at time of the lumpectomy or mastectomy surgery. Doing these prognostic tests on the "entire tumor" rather than on a tiny piece is usually preferred by the pathologist. These two prognostic tests are described here.

The pathologist will look at the cells to determine if they are stimulated to grow by estrogen or progesterone. This will be listed as hormone receptors or "ER" for Estrogen Receptor or "PR" for Progesterone Receptor. Hormone receptors positive means that the cells are stimulated to grow by estrogen or progesterone hormones. This is considered a favorable prognostic factor.

An additional test is called HER2neu receptor. It is done specifically on invasive cancer cells and is not applicable to testing for noninvasive (DCIS) cells. This is an onco-gene measurement. The role of oncogenes is to control cell growth. Extra protein makes cells grow out of control. If the HER2neu test is "positive," then it means that the cancer cells have too much HER2neu receptor protein on the surface of the cell or there are extra copies of the HER2neu gene that can lead to HER2neu overexpression. In some cases, recommendations for special targeted biologic therapy are advised as part of your treatment.

UNDERSTANDING HOW THE STAGE OF YOUR
BREAST CANCER IS DETERMINED

Don't confuse stage with grade. This is a very common mistake. They are quite different. Grade, as just discussed, is related to cell growth. Grade is determined from the biopsy information, but stage requires more details about the cancer and its behavior and measurements. Stage combines several pieces of information (diameter of the invasive portion of the tumor, nodal involvement, and other organ involvement) and is in some degree tied to survival estimates. Remember, however, that you are not a statistic. You are a person. People need to fall on both sides of the statistics to produce these numbers. You are embarking on doing whatever is necessary to be on the survival side.

Stage 0 is noninvasive breast cancer, or DCIS. Cancer cells are limited to the lining of the ducts and have gone no further. The amount of DCIS doesn't need to be measured to determine the stage. Noninvasive disease is always stage 0.

Stage 1 cancer has spread from the ducts or lobules into the nearby fatty tissue of the breast. The tumor diameter is less than 2 cm (less than an inch); there is no cancer in the lymph nodes.

Stage 2 cancer has spread from the ducts or lobules into the nearby fatty tissue of the breast. The tumor diameter is between 2 and 5 cm (1–2 inches); sometimes there is lymph node involvement.

Early-stage breast cancers are considered stages 1 and 2.

In stage 3, the tumor may be larger than 5 cm (2 inches), and the cancer may or may not have spread to the lymph nodes; or the tumor is smaller with evidence of cancer in several lymph nodes. Stage 3 breast cancer is considered locally advanced, and there is a risk that it may also have spread to other organs.

Stage 4 is known as metastatic breast cancer. The cancer has spread from the breast and lymph nodes to other organs in the body, usually the bone, liver, lung, or brain. The presence of cancer in other organs is determined by scans and/or biopsies of these sites, where signs or symptoms were noted.

There are two methods of cancer staging: clinical and pathological. Clinical staging is based on clinical breast examination findings; measurements "guesstimated" on mammograms, ultrasounds, and breast MRIs; examination of the axillae; and other X-rays or scans that may be done. Pathology staging is more precise and is based on the pathologist actually measuring the diameter of the invasive cells once the surgery has been done, looking under the microscope to see if cancer cells are in the lymph nodes, and evaluating other tissue samples that might have been obtained through a biopsy of other organ sites.

GENETICS OF BREAST CANCER

For women with a family history of breast cancer, especially if they are young themselves and their family members were diagnosed premenopausally, the doctor might discuss considering a genetics counseling session. Twelve to 15 percent of women diagnosed have a family history of breast cancer to some degree. When we see multiple family members, especially first-degree relatives, with breast or ovarian cancer, it raises the question of genetics possibly contributing to the underlying cause.

Though it may sound simple to get a blood test to discover the presence of a breast cancer gene (BRCA 1 and BRCA 2 are the two known breast cancer genes that cause breast cancer), it should not be done without genetics counseling and understanding the ramifications of what it means to test positive—as well as what it means to test negative. Additionally, deciding what to do with the results must be factored in. How aggressive would you want to be if you tested positive? Would you consider getting prophylactic (also known as preventive) surgeries to reduce your risk of getting breast cancer? What is the impact this news can have on the next generation? (Fifty percent of children born to a parent carrying one of these genes will also have the gene.) Some people feel guilty if they test negative and their sibling tests positive and vice versa.

Experts anticipate that in the future there will be additional blood tests for other breast cancer genes, so testing negative for BRCA 1 or BRCA 2 isn't a guarantee that genetics are not playing a role in your breast cancer development. Such testing after counseling can be a valuable step in providing information for planning your treatment if you meet criteria for being evaluated for a genetic cause of your breast cancer.

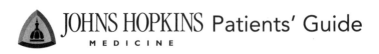

JOHNS HOPKINS Patients' Guide
MEDICINE

MY TEAM—
MEETING YOUR TREATMENT
TEAM

**TEAM MEMBERS—SURGICAL ONCOLOGIST,
MEDICAL ONCOLOGIST, RADIATION ONCOLOGIST,
RADIOLOGIST, PLASTIC SURGEON, PATHOLOGIST,
NURSES, AND OTHERS**

There will be many medical professionals who will make
up your breast cancer oncology team, all with a shared
goal—for you to be well again. Each has a specific role and
specialty related to breast cancer and its treatment. The following is a list of the major members of your team:

Surgical Oncologist. This will be someone who
specializes in breast cancer and performs the
breast cancer surgery—mastectomy, lumpectomy,

sentinel node biopsy, or axillary node dissections. This is usually the first specialist you see.

Medical Oncologist. This is someone who specializes in breast cancer and selects the medicines for your systemic treatment, which may include chemotherapy, hormonal therapy, and/or targeted therapy. The consultation with this doctor is usually after your surgery is completed, about 1–2 weeks postoperative when final pathology results are available.

Radiation Oncologist. This doctor specializes in breast cancer and provides recommendations about radiation therapy.

Radiologist. This doctor may have performed the mammogram as well as the core biopsy to diagnose you. Additional breast imaging studies may be done by this specialist as well.

Plastic Surgeon. For those having mastectomy with reconstruction, this physician specializes in the rebuilding of the breast.

Pathologist. Although you will probably never meet this person, he or she is one of the most important people on your team. The pathologist looks through the microscope at your biopsy tissue and your breast cancer surgery tissue to determine the size of the tumor and whether the cancer is in the lymph nodes, and also provides important prognostic information that is used to determine your treatment plan.

Nurses. There will be several. You will probably meet a new one during each portion of your journey through treatment, beginning with the surgery and followed by chemotherapy, radiation, and long-term care. Educating you, assessing your clinical needs, administering chemotherapy drugs, and evaluating your progress during radiation are some of their functions.

Social Worker. This is someone who specializes in support as well as addressing financial concerns you may have.

Survivor Volunteer. Many breast centers offer emotional support through survivor volunteers who have completed their treatment of breast cancer and want to provide one-on-one support to newly-diagnosed breast cancer patients like you. They provide a candid view of what to expect and can be a great support along your journey.

MAKING YOUR INITIAL APPOINTMENT AT THE BREAST CENTER

The doctor you should be meeting for your first consultation about your breast cancer diagnosis should be a breast surgical oncologist. This is a doctor, mentioned earlier, who specializes in the field of cancer surgery and within that specialty, breast cancer. Many doctors call themselves breast surgeons, but that doesn't mean they are specialists or were trained as such. Knowing their credentials, board certification, the volume of breast cancer patients they treat, and also asking them about some quality measures is useful. You want someone who does more than 100 breast cancer surgeries a year; note, this is more specific than simply saying "breast surgeries." Biopsies are not to be included in these numbers. A good breast surgeon refers patients to a breast radiologist to perform the majority (greater than 90 percent) of breast biopsies that need to be done. So be specific. You have the right to these answers. If the doctor says he or she doesn't know, that may be a signal for you to seek guidance and treatment elsewhere. All physicians know the volume of breast cancer patients they treat. It's not a mystery.

MAKING THE APPOINTMENT

Be sure the person helping to arrange your appointment knows you are newly diagnosed with breast cancer. Even though you may feel differently, this is not an emergency for which you need to be seen in the next day or two. However, most facilities do arrange for patient appointments quite promptly. There are estimates that a speck of breast cancer showing on a mammogram means it has already been growing for several years (there are exceptions, but only a few). This time frame also means you have the necessary time to make good decisions and be sure that you have yourself in capable hands. If the breast center has a website, before making any appointments, you might want to look at it and see if the faculty's biographies are listed and if there is a particular doctor you think you may prefer to see over another.

Be sure to get a specific address and clear directions as to where you are to go and what time you are to report there. If you haven't been to this facility before, allow yourself extra drive time to find it, locate parking, and get to the location where your doctor will be. Being late only frustrates you and your doctor. Arriving early gives you time to sit in the waiting area and review your questions one more time and take in deep breaths so your visit can be as productive as possible.

WHAT TO BRING WITH YOU FOR THAT FIRST CONSULTATION

You've got your appointment and directions where to go and you know what time to arrive. More than likely the scheduler you spoke with also provided instructions regarding what to bring. Just in case the information wasn't clear, the following information will help to ensure that your visit is as productive and efficient as possible for you and the doctor you who will be seeing you.

Bring with you all those X-rays that have been done on your breast to date; this includes mammograms, ultrasounds, and breast MRIs. The doctor may have requested that the pathology slides be shipped in advance with the goal that his or her breast pathologist would be able to look at them prior to your arrival and render an opinion about the accuracy of the information provided in the typed report from the biopsy. Also know in advance if your insurance company requires you to get preauthorization for having additional tests (such as a breast MRI or ultrasound). There are situations in which the doctor finds the films less than satisfactory. When this occurs, she or he may want to get additional imaging done while you are there for this visit. More than likely the doctor will want to have you leave your mammograms and other breast imaging studies there for him or her to review with others (such as a breast imaging radiologist). The facility where they were originally done may have told you that you must bring them back right away. Not so. They are technically your property. The doctor needs to retain them for a time and will use them during your surgical care. Don't feel intimidated if the facility where they were done makes demands that your surgeon says you cannot fulfill. Leave it to his or her office to handle their questions and/or inquiries about when the X-rays will be returned.

WHO TO BRING WITH YOU

Bring a trusted family member or friend with you. When someone is stressed, he or she only hears and retains 10 percent of what is said to him or her. The doctor will be talking a great deal, and you may feel overwhelmed trying to keep it all straight in your mind. The person with you can serve as a scribe. Bring a tape recorder with you as well. Most doctors are very comfortable with the discussion being voice recorded.

WHAT ELSE TO BRING

Be sure to also bring an accurate list of what surgeries you have previously had, what medications you are taking (including vitamins and herbs), what allergies you might have, what other procedures have been done on your breast in the past, and your family history for cancers, heart disease, diabetes, lung disease, and other serious illnesses. If you aren't sure, call another family member and recruit help in obtaining this information because it is important for your medical summary and may influence some decision making about your treatment recommendations.

WHAT QUESTIONS TO ASK DURING YOUR VISIT

Preparing a list of questions in advance is helpful in making the time you have with the doctor as efficient and optimal as possible. The following is a list to help you get started:

1. What type of breast cancer do I have?

2. Did you feel anything in my lymph nodes when you examined me?

3. What stage of disease do you "guesstimate" I have based on what you know so far from my clinical examination, X-rays, and tests?

4. Am I a candidate for lumpectomy or do I need a mastectomy, and how did you make this determination?

5. What surgical method do you use for evaluating my lymph nodes?

6. Did your pathology team confirm the accuracy of the biopsy results?

7. How soon will my surgery be scheduled?

8. What educational information do you offer to prepare me for surgery and for what to expect after surgery?

9. May I speak to a breast cancer survivor volunteer who had the same surgery done here and had a similar treatment plan to what you have planned for me?

10. Who will be my contact for questions I may have?

11. Do you have educational materials for other family members, such as my children?

12. How many breast cancer surgeries do you perform a year?

13. How long have you been in practice doing breast cancer surgeries?

14. Do you have photos I can see of other patients postoperatively to get some idea of what my incision(s) will look like?

15. Who else will be involved in my care, and when will I meet them?

16. How soon after surgery will I see a medical oncologist and/or radiation oncologist?

17. Do you anticipate I will need chemotherapy, and if so, why?

18. Do you anticipate I will need radiation, and if so, why?

19. How often will I be seeing you for ongoing evaluation after my surgery?

20. Are there any clinical trials you would want to recommend for me to consider at this point?

21. Who will be coordinating my care? Do you have a contact person to help me with appointment scheduling and follow-up questions as well as patient education and to help me navigate my breast cancer treatment?

22. How are subsequent appointments arranged for me, and when do these happen?

WHAT TESTS NEED TO BE DONE

For women with what appears to be early stage breast cancer—stage 0, 1, or 2 without clinical evidence of lymph node involvement on clinical examination—no scans are generally done. Scans used to be routine in early stage breast cancer, but they are no longer recommended. Studies have shown that they are not helpful, and are not a good use of your time or of healthcare resources. Scans are done to see if cancer has spread to other organs. If the probability of cancer having spread is slim (a tiny stage 1 tumor, for example), then it would be inappropriate to get a bone scan or CAT scan. On the other hand, if a woman presents with a large tumor and palpable lymph nodes in her armpit area, scans are done to assess whether the disease has already spread elsewhere. Additionally, if she has a tumor with unfavorable prognostic factors and has complaints of back pain, hip pain, headaches, or other symptoms that have lingered for several weeks without explanation to their cause, scans may be done.

After reviewing your mammograms or other breast imaging studies, your surgeon may decide that additional studies are necessary to provide greater detail about the breast tissue and where the cancer is located. Don't be surprised or caught off guard by this possibility. You want your surgeon to be thorough. Remember, your doctor has your best interest at heart.

Although blood tests are usually not done for early stage breast cancers, your surgeon may include some as part of your routine preoperative evaluation. You may also need to have a chest X-ray and EKG. These are not tests specifically related to a diagnosis of cancer but instead are done routinely on anyone having an operation.

HOW BEST TO CONTACT TEAM MEMBERS

Request business cards from each healthcare provider you see, and ask what their office procedure is for responding to questions or concerns you may have. Usually there is one contact person to serve this role. Find out also if you are at liberty to communicate with any of the team by email. If and when questions arise, be succinct and think all your thoughts through. It is better to ask three questions at once than one question three different times to three different healthcare providers.

NAVIGATING APPOINTMENTS

Some breast centers have people to assist you who are referred to as patient navigators. The term navigator is loosely defined, though, and sometimes is used strictly for marketing, in which case the person does not really navigate patients through their medical journey. Therefore, when you inquire about this service, describe the tasks you anticipate needing help with. Ask about the process for assisting you with appointment scheduling, getting test results back, getting scheduled for surgery, seeing a medical oncologist and possibly the radiation oncologist after your surgery, and in general having someone available for support and to address any other clinical needs that may arise. In some cases, your point person may be a nurse in the breast center or an office manager in the doctor's office. In other cases, it may be a navigator or case manager. The title isn't important but the functions are.

FINANCIAL IMPLICATIONS OF TREATMENT/ INSURANCE CLEARANCE

You didn't plan on getting diagnosed with breast cancer. No doubt this was never one of your goals to have to be addressing for yourself. There is no convenient time to get this disease, and the diagnosis alone can wreak havoc in your life. If you are working outside the home, you will be taking time off for your surgery and possibly for other treatments. Getting your ducks in a row early is smart. Learning how much sick leave you have, your short-term disability coverage, copayment information, prescription coverage, and other medical expense issues is helpful for planning your budget, which will be changing for a short while. Your insurance company may require referrals to be obtained in order to see certain specialists, get tests done, and get surgery authorized, as well as other treatments. If you need help with these things, ask for a social worker to assist you. Some breast centers also have financial assistants to help you.

There may be some treatments that are recommended that relate to clinical trials. Some may be covered by your insurance while others may not. If you are interested in participating in a clinical trial, a research nurse will help get you this information.

If you lack health insurance, all is not lost. There are resources available for women who need help and meet certain criteria for financial assistance and coverage of their breast cancer treatment expenses. Some states even have special grants for residents for precisely this purpose. Check with the social worker at the facility where you are being treated to get assistance and referrals. There are also organizations that provide transportation to and from treatment visits, provide food for you and your family, and even assist with coverage of some medications. They aren't available in every state, so rely on your social worker to tell you more about what is available for your geographic area.

Financial support services are not well advertised. It will require you to take the initiative to ask about them rather than waiting for someone to tell you about them. Be assertive and do this for yourself. That's why these programs exist. Money is the primary reason family members get into arguments. Avoid this upfront by discussing the issue and planning a budget. Be proactive in asking to meet with the social worker to discuss what support services are available for you as well.

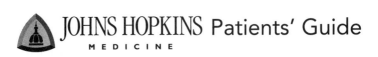

CHAPTER 3

JOHNS HOPKINS Patients' Guide
MEDICINE

TAKING ACTION—
COMPREHENSIVE TREATMENT
CONSIDERATIONS

This chapter will describe each of the various phases of treatment and the decision making involved in determining the best treatment for you. Breast cancer treatment can include surgery, chemotherapy, radiation therapy, hormonal therapy, and targeted therapy. Some women need all of these therapies; others just need one or two. The number of therapies doesn't always match up with the severity of the disease. Let's review each one.

SURGICAL TREATMENT

Society associates women's breasts with beauty, femininity, sexiness, and motherhood. Society admires cleavage and promotes it. Breast cancer surgery can threaten a woman's self-image. She may fear that she will feel like less of a woman and may worry even more that her partner will feel differently about her sexually. Talking through this very important issue is critical and should take place before surgery.

The majority of women today have surgical options of lumpectomy, mastectomy, or mastectomy with breast reconstruction. The survival rate is equal for lumpectomy with radiation and mastectomy. Factors that influence the possibility and advisability of these options are the size and location of the tumor, type of breast cancer, size of the woman's breast, possibly the age of the woman at time of diagnosis, and other prognostic factors, as well as her general health. A woman with a large tumor compared to her breast volume usually is advised to do mastectomy surgery. (Sometimes chemotherapy given before surgery shrinks the tumor enough to permit lumpectomy.) Someone with multiple tumors that occupy several different quadrants of the breast will usually be told that she is not a good candidate for breast-conserving surgery.

It's important to restate that survival is equal whether lumpectomy (with radiation) or mastectomy is done as the surgical treatment. Risk of recurrence is slightly different, but you should not use it as the major factor to decide what type of surgical treatment you choose. For women undergoing lumpectomy and radiation, risk of recurrence usually is around 10 percent. This is *local recurrence*, meaning the breast cancer recurred in the breast where it once was before. For women undergoing mastectomy surgery, the risk of local recurrence is around 1–2 percent. Ten percent may sound like a large number but it really is not. Turn that percentage around: 90 percent of women do not develop a recurrence, and even those who do are likely to survive just as long as they would have without such a recurrence. Therefore, the majority of women choose breast conserving—lumpectomy with radiation—when given this option.

CONSIDERING BREAST RECONSTRUCTION

Women undergoing mastectomy usually have options about whether they wish to have breast reconstruction. Although the decision is a personal one, it is usually made with a great deal of input from the woman's partner. If reconstruction is an option, the surgeon will refer you to a plastic surgeon for consultation. At this point, you should be given an opportunity to review photos (torso shots) of women who have had various forms of reconstruction. Some breast centers have survivor volunteers available who can talk candidly with you about their personal experiences with the reconstruction process.

Reconstruction options include breast implants or moving fat and tissue from one part of the body to the chest to rebuild your breast. Most women are candidates for some type of reconstruction. The timing and specific type of reconstruction recommended depend on the stage and aggressiveness of the disease, the amount of fatty tissue you have, your medical history, whether radiation is needed after surgery, and your own body image.

There is no right or wrong answer about breast reconstruction. Each woman, with input from those she trusts, needs to decide this for herself. You may have assumptions about the way you feel about your breasts that surprise you. Because surgery is usually the first step of treatment, it is important to express your feelings and work through them.

Women commonly want to rush through treatment and not do reconstruction. They are so focused on survival that they shortchange themselves. It has been said that women need permission to choose to pursue reconstruction. Reconstruction doesn't delay your treatment or affect your long-term survival outcome. It also doesn't make it more difficult to diagnose a recurrence if it were to happen. These are common worries of newly-diagnosed patients, however. Explore your options and think about how you want to look and feel a year from now. Don't focus solely on rushing through the process. A short-term investment of time now to consider reconstruction can be one of the most important things you do for yourself along this journey of treatment. Don't worry about insurance coverage for this. Thanks to the Women's Health and Cancer Rights Act passed in October 1998, reconstruction is covered by your health insurance.

Women who desire immediate reconstruction but, for medical reasons, are not good candidates for the procedure need to find peace within themselves about this situation. Talking with other breast cancer survivors who have experienced the same situation can be very enlightening and useful. Your healthcare team can connect you with a local support group. In most cases, reconstruction can be at the end of treatment and may give you something to look forward to later. Until then, consider yourself a "work in progress," like an oil painting masterpiece.

TYPES OF BREAST CANCER SURGERY

The following are types of breast cancer surgery that may be discussed with you as potential options:

Lumpectomy. This is the removal of the tumor in the breast with a margin of healthy tissue around it in all six directions; also known as a breast-conserving surgery or partial mastectomy. Recovery time is usually just a few days.

Sentinel Node Biopsy. The sentinel node biopsy involves the identification and surgical removal of the sentinel lymph node. Lymph nodes serve as a filtering system for the lymphatic system (a system of vessels that collects fluids from cells for filtrating). The sentinel node is also known as the guard node. It is considered the first node in the armpit area (also known as the axillae) that would be affected by cancer; this means if the cancer were to spread from the breast to the axillary nodes, it would go to this specific node first. This node is identified either by use of a special blue dye or by use of radioactive isotope injected into the breast before the surgery is begun. This procedure for identification of the sentinel node is also known as sentinel node mapping. Both methods of identifying the sentinel node are considered highly accurate. It is the surgeon's option which method is used based on his or her training and expertise. The node is then sent to pathology to determine if there is cancer in this node. (Occasionally, there will be several nodes that are identified to be the sentinel node. When this occurs, all identified sentinel nodes are removed and sent for pathology to evaluate. This could be two or three nodes but usually not more than that.) If there is no cancer in the sentinel node, then the rest of the nodes can be left alone because the risk of there being cancer in other nodes is extremely low. This procedure, now a standard of care, dramatically reduces the risk of lymphedema and other arm problems associated with a full axillary node dissection. A separate, very small incision, just below the hair line in your armpit, is made to access and identify the sentinel node and surgically remove it. (For women having a mastectomy, in some cases it may be accessible without a separate incision.) If the sentinel node does contain cancer, then an axillary node dissection is done.

Axillary Node Dissection. This is done if the sentinel node is found to contain cancer cells or if breast imaging studies (such as ultrasound or other X-rays or scans) show an enlarged node that a biopsy found to contain cancer cells. An axillary node dissection is the surgical removal of the lymph nodes in the armpit area. There are three levels of nodes (level 1, 2, and 3). These levels are anatomically found in the armpit area. If cancer were found in the sentinel node, then usually level 1 and 2 node dissections are done, leaving level 3 intact. (Gone are the days of removing all the lymph nodes.) The pathology results from an axillary node dissection help to plan the staging information of the disease so that the number of nodes containing cancer is known. This is important for planning additional treatment including chemotherapy and radiation. This procedure is generally done as an outpatient surgery procedure (unless done as part of a mastectomy procedure that involves reconstruction). A drain is usually inserted and will remain in for several days. The risk of lymphedema increases when there is a need to dissect these additional nodes. Getting instructions about ways to reduce this risk is important and should be reviewed with you prior to your surgery. Most women who have axillary node dissections do not ever develop lymphedema, however. Range of motion and arm strength usually is regained in 2–3 weeks.

Total Simple Mastectomy. This is the removal of the breast, nipple, and areola. A sentinel node biopsy might be performed at the same time. Recovery from this procedure, if no reconstruction is done at the same time, is usually 1–2 weeks. Hospitalization varies; for some, it may be an outpatient procedure and for others it may require an overnight stay. A drain is usually inserted that is removed several days later and is easy to take care of at home.

Modified Radical Mastectomy. This procedure involves removal of the breast, nipple, and areola, as well as an axillary node dissection. Recovery, when surgery is done without reconstruction, is usually 3–4 weeks.

Skin-Sparing Mastectomy. This is the removal of the breast, nipple, and areola, but the outer skin of the breast is kept intact. It is a special method of performing a mastectomy (total simple or modified radical) that allows for good cosmetic outcome when combined with reconstruction done at the same time. There are special circumstances when the nipple and/or areola can also be saved, but this is not commonly done, recognizing that leaving behind breast tissue may increase the risk of local recurrence. There also is no sensation in the nipple if it is "saved."

Breast Implant Reconstruction. Usually done at the time of the mastectomy surgery, a tissue expander is placed underneath the chest muscle, and over a period of several weeks, it is expanded by injecting sterile water into it, thus stretching it like a balloon. Once it has reached the expansion size desired, the tissue expander is removed and replaced with a permanent implant. Implants can be silicone, saline, or a combination of both. Hospitalization usually is overnight, and recovery takes 2–3 weeks. There is some discomfort with the expansion process because it is stretching the chest muscle.

TRAM (Transverse Rectus Abdominis Myocutaneous) Flap Reconstruction. This is a procedure taking the tummy tissue and fat along with the muscle that provides the blood supply and tunneling the tissue to the chest to rebuild the breast, forming a breast-shaped mound. Hospitalization is commonly 4–6 nights and recovery is 6–8 weeks due to the moving of the muscle. There is a risk of abdominal hernia later with this method due to muscle loss. If done bilaterally (both sides), the risk of abdominal hernia can be higher. Women receiving this reconstruction are discouraged from short- and long-term heavy lifting. This procedure results in a tummy tuck.

Latissimus Dorsi Flap Reconstruction. This procedure takes the tissue, fat, and muscle from under the shoulder blade and brings it to the front to rebuild the breast. Hospitalization is 3–5 days and the recovery period is 5–6 weeks. Some women later report difficulty doing rigorous exercise that involves this muscle, such as swimming or golfing. As with all procedures, factor your lifestyle into your decision about the type of reconstruction to consider.

DIEP (Deep Inferior Epigastric Perforator) Flap Reconstruction. This surgery involves taking tummy tissue and fat but no muscle. The doctor must identify one of the tiny blood vessels in the muscle; tease it out of the muscle, leaving the muscle wall intact; cut the tissue free from the body; and transplant the tissue and fat to the chest to rebuild the breast. It requires a microvascular procedure to reconnect the blood vessel in the chest area. This is a highly technical procedure that requires a microscope to reconnect the vascular supply. Hospitalization is 3–4 days; recovery is 4–5 weeks. There are no long-term lifting restrictions since the muscle was not sacrificed. This is a procedure considered superior to doing the TRAM flap. However, only a few breast centers have plastic surgeons with expertise in this procedure. It is worth traveling the distance to have the surgery done in order to benefit from this improved technique that carries low risk of hernia and avoids lifting restrictions. It too results in a tummy tuck.

S-GAP (Superior Gluteal Artery Perforator) Flap Reconstruction. This reconstruction method uses the gluteal fat from the buttocks to rebuild the breast. It requires microvascular surgery to reconnect the blood vessels. Hospitalization is 3–4 days and recovery usually takes 3–4 weeks. This surgery is not commonly done, and again requires an experienced plastic surgeon who specializes in this type of procedure. For women not interested in implants or who for some reason are not a candidate for them and lack abdominal fat as well, this can be a very nice option.

Oncoplastic Surgery. This is a relatively new term. It means that the patient is undergoing lumpectomy surgery and will have the breast reshaped, along with possibly reducing the other breast in size to maintain symmetry. There are also some situations in which the breast may undergo a large lumpectomy and an implant will

be added to help accommodate for lost volume.
The first scenario is the more common, however.

Nipple Reconstruction. This procedure is
generally done several months after the breast
reconstruction so that the tissue/implant has
"settled in." This waiting helps ensure accurate
placement of the nipple. It is done as an outpatient
procedure, and the breast mound is used to create
the nipple. The eyes seek symmetry, so every
effort is made on the part of the plastic surgeon
to "match" the nipple construction with that
of the natural nipple on the other breast. This
reconstructed nipple will not have sensation
or a change in appearance from stimulation
or temperature change. No real recovery time
is needed. Local anesthetic is given for the
procedure. No compression of the newly-built
nipple is to be done for 2 weeks, to avoid causing
it to flatten while it heals. (If the patient is
undergoing bilateral nipple reconstruction, then
she can discuss with the plastic surgeon the type
of nipples she wants to have and the amount of
projection she is seeking since she has the option
and doesn't need to match the remaining nipple.)

Areola Tattooing. Organic tattoo dye is used to
create an areola. This is commonly done by a
nurse practitioner or physician's assistant in the
plastic surgeon's office. The diameter and pallet
shade is matched to the remaining breast. If the
patient is undergoing bilateral areola tattooing,
then she can choose her diameter and color. This

procedure takes approximately 30–40 minutes per side. There can be some fading of the color, requiring it to be touched up later in some cases. No recovery time is needed, but keeping it dry and clean during the healing process is important. Women are discouraged from going to a tattoo parlor to have this done, because the tattoo dye substance is different. Dyes in tattoo parlors contain lead that could appear as an abnormality on a future MRI if one needed to be done.

Once the decision is finally made about what surgical treatment is best for you, you will feel better. You now will be taking action against the disease. No matter what surgical option is selected, on the day of surgery, focus on this being your "transformation day": You are being transformed from a breast cancer victim into a breast cancer survivor and taking your first leap up the survival curve by ridding your body of the source of this disease.

SOME INFORMATION ABOUT DRAINS AND EXTERNAL PROSTHESIS

Mastectomy surgeries as well as axillary node dissection and reconstruction usually involve the placement of small drains. These are left in for several days. One of the nurses in the breast center will show you how to care for your drains and incisions during your recovery process. Pertinent exercises will also be demonstrated to get range of motion and body strength back as soon as possible.

If you are embarking on a mastectomy without reconstruction, you usually will be eligible to be fitted for a breast prosthesis 6–8 weeks after your surgery. During the interim, the doctor will give you a temporary lightweight breast form to wear inside a surgical bra. When going to be fitted for your breast prosthesis, seek out a mastectomy supply shop that has a certified fitter. A proper-fitting mastectomy bra and prosthesis are important for balance, comfort, and confidence.

ACCEPTING HELP AT HOME

Deciding who will help you at home after surgery sounds simple but sometimes isn't. You may need some assistance at home managing drains for a few days, attending to wound care and such, and recovering from surgery in general. The length of time you need help will depend on the type of surgery you have. Ask the surgeon what to expect, and request to meet with your nurse to review teaching instructions preoperatively so you are well prepared as to what to expect.

If other people will be coming to stay to help you, talk about roles and responsibilities beforehand. Write out what each person is responsible for doing—buying the groceries, changing bandages, making dinner, taking the kids to soccer practice, and so on. Planning ahead prevents problems later. Function as a team—remember, this is a team effort! You and your family member or friend who will be helping to take care of you need to talk about your expectations of each other.

If your surgery involves drains and wound management at home, decide in advance who will be responsible for helping with emptying the drains and providing the dressing

changes. Again, photographs of what to expect are helpful. For women having a lumpectomy, there will usually
be little difference in the overall appearance of the breast.
Women undergoing mastectomy without reconstruction
will look like a young girl again, with a smooth flat chest on
one side. For women undergoing reconstruction, it will be
important to look at the surgical site as a work in progress.
Reconstruction takes several weeks to take shape and also
may require additional surgery for the final cosmetic result
to be completed.

RESUMING PHYSICAL INTIMACY AFTER SURGERY

No matter what type of surgery you had performed, shortly
after you are home from the hospital, your doctor will in-
struct you to do a specific set of exercises to begin regain-
ing arm strength, range of motion, and general physical
well-being. If you have had flap reconstruction, there will
be additional exercises to regain abdominal strength and
motion. A nice way to begin resuming closeness is to have
your partner help you with your arm exercises. A slow
dance and some romantic music are perfect for this purpose. Consider it part of your exercise routine. During your
first song, you may have your hands resting on his shoul-
ders and by the third song, they are up and crossed around
his neck.

The timing of when the doctor says you can resume sexual
activities will vary depending on the type of surgery you
have. The time frame is usually quite short for women undergoing lumpectomy or mastectomy without reconstruction. With reconstructive surgery, however, ask your plastic

surgeon about which physical activities—including sex—can be resumed and when.

Your body—and most specifically one of your erogenous zones—has experienced a change. Get to know your body again, and let your partner explore this with you. Your partner may be at a loss for words and not know what to say. He may wonder if it is okay to touch your incision; he doesn't want to cause discomfort. Let your partner know what you want. Being silent usually is not helpful.

ADJUSTING TO YOUR ALTERED BODY IMAGE

One issue that a woman who has undergone mastectomy surgery might encounter is deciding when to actually look at the incision. The woman, as the patient, needs to be in charge of that decision. Some women are comfortable right away; others delay for some time. Don't delay too long though. It is advisable to talk about this with your partner in advance and agree on a plan. Looking at photographs together in the doctor's office can help, too, to know what to expect.

ADJUVANT TREATMENT AFTER SURGERY

The need for additional treatment in the form of chemotherapy, radiation therapy, targeted biologic therapy, or hormonal therapy will depend on the stage of the disease, type of surgery performed, the grade of the cancer cells, the age of the patient, the general health of the patient, and other prognostic factors determined by the pathologist after examining the tumor obtained from surgery. It is routine and should be expected that women undergoing lumpectomy surgery will need radiation therapy of the conserved breast to help ensure that the cancer doesn't return. The need for chemotherapy, however, is unrelated to the type of surgery done; it is based on the degree of risk of the cancer returning in a distant organ site. Hormonal therapy is recommended about 50 percent of the time to patients as a means of reducing the risk of recurrence of breast cancer for women whose cancer cells were hormone receptor positive.

When you look at the entire treatment experience from beginning to end for women needing surgery, chemotherapy, and radiation, it lasts, on average, about 9 months—the same length of time it takes to conceive and give birth to a child. That is the best way to look at your breast cancer treatment, too—you are being reborn a healthier woman with the goal to become cancer-free.

CHEMOTHERAPY

Many different chemotherapy drugs are available today for treating breast cancer and preventing its return. Though usually this type of treatment happens after surgery, there are exceptions. The following information explains more about this type of treatment and what to expect.

NEOADJUVANT CHEMOTHERAPY

There are special circumstances in which chemotherapy is actually recommended as the first phase of treatment against breast cancer. In such cases, it is referred to as neoadjuvant chemotherapy and is given prior to the patient undergoing surgery. The mission of the chemotherapy in such cases is to carry medicine to all parts of the body where the disease may be located, including beyond the breast itself. This may be recommended for women with locally advanced disease in which it is known that the lymph nodes contain cancer, therefore increasing the risk of disease potentially having spread elsewhere. Women with relatively large breast tumors, or women with relatively average-size tumors who are smaller breasted and hoping for lumpectomy surgery, may be advised to do chemotherapy first, unrelated to their nodal status. The chemotherapy is given to hopefully shrink the tumor, thus increasing the likelihood of the patient being able to have less surgery than originally anticipated.

CHEMOTHERAPY GIVEN AFTER SURGERY

The medical oncologist will determine if you will need chemotherapy based on information learned by pathology from the surgery that was recently completed. For women with early stage breast cancer, the prognostic factors from the surgical pathology strongly impact this decision. Patients with small tumors that are hormone receptor positive and HER2neu negative may fall into a "gray zone" for whether chemotherapy would be of benefit. Therefore, risks and benefits of doing chemotherapy are carefully weighed. A pathology test called Oncotype DX might be recommended to be done on the cancer cells to help provide additional information about the behavior and characteristics of the tumor and the likelihood of this specific cancer recurring in the future. The test provides a score regarding this probability. Patients with a low score are usually told that chemotherapy may not be that beneficial, given the low probability of the cancer returning; those with a high score are usually encouraged to take chemotherapy. Patients with a score in the intermediate group have longer discussions about the pros and cons of chemotherapy.

Age, too, is a factor in deciding for whom chemotherapy is appropriate. Elderly, frail patients, for example, may be advised that chemotherapy would not be wise for them. Someone young, say in her early 30s, with an aggressive tumor would probably be advised to take it as part of her treatment plan.

Stage of the disease, grade of the cells, hormone receptor status, HER2neu receptor status, and some other clinical and pathology factors influence this decision-making process. There is no "one right answer" that serves everyone.

How much of a worrier a patient is can also influence this decision. A patient who is told her survival benefit is increased by 3 percent by taking chemotherapy may consider that too low a number to make it worth her while. Another patient who is told the same thing may say that she wants to do it even if the benefit were only 1 percent. It's a personal choice. It is important though to be educated about the risks and benefits so that you can make logical and thoughtful decisions with the medical oncologist as your adviser.

SIDE EFFECTS OF CHEMOTHERAPY

Chemotherapy, a form of systemic treatment, can cause a second wave of distress due to probable hair loss, gastrointestinal symptoms, and fatigue. Chemotherapy usually is administered intravenously and given to patients in an outpatient setting. Some protocols call for a cycle of treatment every 3 weeks; others may be more frequent. Most women undergoing chemotherapy will have treatments given over a 3- to 6-month period.

Most chemotherapy regimens for breast cancer cause hair loss during treatment. Preparing in advance for this is helpful. For some women, this experience is more traumatic than losing part or all of their breast. Women recognize that their hair is visible to all who see them and is also something they may take particular pride in. Seeing a bald woman tells society that they are looking at someone "with cancer." Some suggestions for managing hair loss are listed here:

- Have a hair stylist cut your hair short about 10 days after your first chemotherapy treatment. (This is usually a day or two before your hair will start coming out on its own. It usually falls out within 24 hours once it starts.)

- Have a "coming-out" party for your hair—everyone brings a hat or other head covering (scarf, turban, etc.). This is a great project for children to do and helps engage family members in the preparation. Consider it similar to a baby shower but the baby is your head instead.

- If you plan to wear a wig, go to be fitted prior to starting chemotherapy. Take someone along with you whom you trust to give you honest feedback regarding how you look. Matching your hair color and style will be easier if you go before chemotherapy starts. (Some patients, however, opt to have a different hair color and style, since this is an opportunity for a "new look.")

• Some women choose to do a buzz cut in advance of hair loss, truly taking control of this situation. They don't want the chemotherapy to control when their hair is gone; they will determine its fate. Wearing a turban or scarf is also an option, as is simply being bald. It is your choice. During the winter months, however, wear knitted caps while outdoors or exposed to the elements. A person loses 80 percent of their body heat from the top of their head. You need to stay bundled up and warm.

• Some insurance companies will cover the expenses for a wig, up to a certain amount (usually around $350). It must be submitted on a prescription as a "skull prosthesis" by your medical oncologist, so make sure to inquire about this.

Talk with the medical oncologist about what steps can be taken to reduce possible side effects from chemotherapy. Today, not everyone experiences side effects. Medications are available to prevent or dramatically reduce nausea; not all chemotherapy drugs cause hair loss. In addition, exercise has been proven to help reduce the side effect of fatigue. (See Chapter 4 for more information.)

FOCUS ON THE POSITIVES

Focus on what chemotherapy is designed to do *for* you— destroy any cancer cells that have spread elsewhere in the body. Use visual imagery to picture how these drugs work, and focus on those images when receiving the drugs.

Most patients feel well the day of the treatment. If side effects are to occur, they most commonly happen the night following chemotherapy or the next day. Celebrate the completing of each cycle of treatment. Remember you are climbing further up the survival curve by taking chemotherapy. Take pride in this victory. It's important to realize that some patients may react differently to chemotherapy than others do. Talking with other breast cancer survivors who have had the same chemotherapy drugs will not answer the question for you on how you personally are going to feel and what side effects you may experience.

Don't select your treatment regimen based on which drugs do or don't cause hair loss either. You want to take the advice of your doctor in helping to decide which drugs will be the right ones for you. There may be several treatment regimens from which you are to choose. You want to know which chemotherapy drugs work best for you and your situation. Your medical oncologist will review your drug options with you based on the prognostic factors learned from your pathology as well as from any scans he or she may have done in advance of starting your treatment. Drugs are commonly given in combination, so you may be receiving several drugs at the same time.

PRECAUTIONS DURING CHEMOTHERAPY

During your chemotherapy, your blood will be taken at designated intervals to make sure your red blood cells and white blood cells are staying within normal limits. If they are low, which is a common side effect, the doctor might decide to give you special medicines to boost your blood counts back up to a normal range.

Be aware of people around you who have a cold or the flu because your immune system is being taxed during the chemotherapy process. Be especially careful of little children who look healthy but may be germ carriers.

The majority of women today continue to work while receiving chemotherapy. Receiving chemotherapy on a Friday, then resting up over the weekend with the help of family and friends has worked for many.

Anticipate that your doctor will discuss the clinical trials for which you may be a candidate. Clinical trials are research studies in which people agree to try new therapies under careful supervision in order to help doctors identify the best treatments with the fewest side effects. These studies help improve the overall standard of care for the future. Clinical trials may provide you an edge over standard treatment and in the future may actually become the new method of treatment for women diagnosed with breast cancer after you.

Remember, too, that there is a beginning and an end to taking chemotherapy. You can deal with anything when you know it is for a designated period of time.

RADIATION

For patients undergoing lumpectomy surgery, or if pathology results confirm there are cancer cells in several lymph nodes, or if the breast tumor itself was large, radiation will probably be recommended after surgery. Radiation is designed to prevent your breast (or the area where your breast or lymph nodes were) from developing breast cancer again and is highly effective in doing its job. Women having lumpectomy without radiation can have as high as a 40 percent risk of recurrence within 2 years. By doing radiation, that risk is reduced to about 10 percent, so consider radiation an important part of your treatment plan if it is recommended that you have it. Radiation is usually done after chemotherapy for those who need that type of systemic treatment.

There have been vast improvements in radiation therapy, also known as local treatment, over the last decade or so. Special technology is used so that only tissues that need to be irradiated are irradiated. Also, although there is some risk of radiation side effects for the heart and lung tissue, this risk is markedly less today than it was years ago. If your breast cancer is in the left breast, however, you will want additional precautions taken to help protect your heart and lungs.

For women undergoing lumpectomy, radiation may make the breast a little pink or puffy. Some women comment that their breast is tender in a way that is similar to premenstrual tenderness. Treatments are daily, Monday through Friday, for usually 5–6 weeks. Although it means going every day to the radiation facility, you are in and out quickly, usually in less than half an hour.

Radiation doesn't hurt. It feels similar to getting a chest X-ray, which means you feel nothing at all. However, radiation is cumulative; that's why you may start getting fatigued toward the last few weeks of treatment. Exercising regularly, such as power walking, has proven to reduce this specific side effect.

The breast area, chest wall, and axillary area are exposed during radiation therapy treatments, but you are behind closed doors with just your treatment team looking in on you. Before radiation begins, you will have some special measurements done, called simulation, to ensure that the radiation beams are lined up the exact same way to irradiate the same area consistently and precisely. A few tiny tattoo marks (little blue dots) will be made on your chest as part of the preparation process. These dots are usually permanent. Some women have become creative once treatment is completed and use the dots as a center of an artistic tattoo such as a butterfly, pink ribbon, or some other symbol of significance to them. Just as your incision is a battle scar of courage, so are these tiny tattoo dots. Do not have these dots taken off later. They are important markings for the future in the event of recurrence or other medical issues related to your heart or lungs.

CLINICAL TRIALS

There are some ongoing clinical trials for doing radiation a bit differently than the traditional external beam radiation. These studies include accelerated radiation, in which the patient receives radiation twice a day for about 2 weeks. Brachytherapy is also being used in studies; this involves the insertion of a balloon during the lumpectomy surgery. Radiation is placed inside the balloon and the breast is irradiated just where the cancer originally was located, along with a margin of healthy tissue around it. This process takes 1 week. There are pros and cons to each method for you to discuss with your radiation oncologist. If you have breast cancer in your left breast and will be undergoing radiation, inquire what steps will be taken to protect your heart and lungs. There are clinical trials today such as the ABC study (active breath control device) that times your breathing with the radiation being given so that your heart and lungs are as far away from radiation exposure as possible.

SUBTLE EFFECTS OF RADIATION

For some women, the effects of radiation can last quite some time with the breast going through subtle changes for as long as a year after treatment is completed. It may feel firmer and be tanner looking or puffy for an extended period of time, or it may even shrink a little.

If a woman has an implant in place, radiation may cause the implant to react in such a way that it becomes hard or feels tighter. The tissue around the implant may shrink causing what is called capsulitis. This may require surgical revisions later by a plastic surgeon. If the patient has undergone mastectomy surgery and has a tissue expander in place, it is advisable to have the radiation, if needed, done while the expander is still there and let it take the radiation hit, then post-radiation, replace it with the permanent implant.

HORMONAL THERAPY

Your medical oncologist will determine if it will be helpful for you to take hormonal therapy. Hormonal therapy is totally different than hormone replacement therapy. Hormonal therapy, in the form of a SERM (selective estrogen receptor modulator) or AIs (aromatase inhibitors), helps disable estrogen from reaching a breast cancer cell or breast cell that wants to mutate into a breast cancer cell in the future. If the pathologist determined that your breast cancer was hormone receptor positive for estrogen and/or progesterone, then anticipate a discussion about taking hormonal therapy. Hormonal therapy is oftentimes the last portion of treatment. It is given after surgery, chemotherapy, and radiation are completed. There are some circumstances in which it may be given prior to the start of any treatments, as a way to help shrink a large breast cancer tumor for a patient who would benefit from chemotherapy given first but for medical reasons isn't able to receive chemotherapy (very elderly patients, for example).

For women whose cancer tested positive for hormone receptors, the doctor would know that hormones in your body may promote growth of breast cancer cells. By giving you a medication that blocks those hormones, the recurrence of the disease usually can be prevented. By taking a drug that works on breast cancer cells like an estrogen blocker, the risk of cancer recurring or possibly continuing to grow is reduced. The treatment is in the form of a pill that is taken daily for 5–10 years. Side effects are similar to menopause. There are also some other side effects that you may experience that your doctor will discuss with you (see Chapter 4).

Hormonal therapy is a long-term commitment on your part. Due to the rapid developments researchers are making in hormonal therapy, you may be advised to take some form of hormonal therapy for a period of time, then switch to a different type for an additional period of time. When a woman is dealing with side effects from taking a medication, there can be issues with adherence to the daily schedule of taking the drug as prescribed. Speak up and make your oncologist aware of any side effects you are experiencing that are causing you to consider discontinuing the medication or self-adjust the dosage. The dosage and frequency for taking the medication has been determined based on extensive research. Altering this schedule may affect the benefit you are (or aren't) receiving from this therapy. Its purpose is to reduce the risk of recurrence of this disease for you. Medications or other over-the-counter treatments can be used to counteract some of these side effects (such as the use of vaginal lubricants for vaginal dryness).

SERM drugs like Nolvadex (tamoxifen) are bone friendly but may cause other side effects that warrant discussion. If you are a smoker, for example, you may be at increased risk for blood clots that could even lead to stroke. AIs like Arimidex (anastrozole), Femara (letrozole), or Aromasin (exemestane), on the other hand, are not bone friendly, and if you are advised to take an AI, talk with your doctor about getting a bone density test done and the frequency with which it should be repeated. It's important to maintain your bone health, so being proactive in measuring it and taking a medicine that builds bone also may be important for you.

TARGETED BIOLOGICAL THERAPY

In recent years, clinical trials have been completed that evaluated the effect of targeted biological therapy. A prognostic factor that was discussed earlier (see Chapter 1) is called the HER2neu receptor. HER2neu stands for human epidermal growth receptor 2. It is a gene that helps control how cells grow, divide, and repair themselves. The HER2neu gene directs the production of special proteins that are called HER2neu receptors. Each healthy breast cell contains two copies of the HER2neu gene. This gene is designed to help cells grow normally. If a cell, however, has too many copies of the HER2neu gene, it can result in too much HER2neu protein being produced. This may result in the normal breast cell turning into a cancer cell. It may also make the cancer cells more aggressive

It's important to not confuse this gene with the BRCA 1 and 2 genes, which may indicate a person's genetic predisposition to develop breast cancer (see Chapter 1).

The pathologist determines with special testing procedures on the invasive breast cancer cells whether the cancer is HER2neu positive or negative. A test result of 0, 1+, or 2+ is considered negative; a result of 3+ is considered positive. Women whose cancers are HER2neu positive (3+) may be candidates for targeted biologic therapy in the form of a drug called Herceptin (trastuzumab). It is antibody therapy, so it works differently than chemotherapy drugs. It works in three different ways: It may block tumor cell growth, it may target the cell for destruction by the immune system itself, or it may work with chemotherapy (paclitaxel) to destroy the HER2neu positive cancer cells. This drug may be given alone or with chemotherapy. When Herceptin is used with chemotherapy that attacks and damages the DNA at the cellular level, Herceptin stops the cells from repairing themselves. Because the cells can't repair themselves, they die.

It is usually recommended that this drug be taken for year and that it be administered weekly. It is given by IV. Blood work as well as heart function tests are done periodically while taking this form of therapy. There is some risk to developing heart problems; therefore, patients are carefully monitored for this.

A second form of biologic targeted therapy is Tykerb (laptinib). It is now approved for women who have developed a resistance to Herceptin. A unique feature of this drug is that it crosses the blood-brain barrier, an important feature for women who have stage IV disease that has spread to their brain. It is taken by pill each day. A third drug in this family of therapies is Avastin (bevacizumab). It is given for women who are HER2neu negative and are battling metastatic disease.

This is a growing area for research and an exciting time to see progress toward altering cell behavior as a way to treat or control breast cancer growth. Because they are "smart drugs" that focus on molecular and cellular changes that are specific to cancer, targeted cancer therapies may be more effective than traditional chemotherapy and less harmful to normal cells. It may become the new way of treating many other cancers in addition to breast cancer.

CLINICAL TRIALS

New and innovative treatments are developed and implemented by doing clinical trials. Without clinical trials, doctors could not improve the treatment of breast cancer, nor could ways be developed to prevent it in the future. They are the backbone of science today. Your doctors may at any given time during your treatment discuss with you opportunities to participate in a clinical trial. Be open minded. Hear what is being offered as part of a study.

There are many different kinds of clinical trials. They range from studies focusing on ways to prevent, detect, diagnose, treat, and control breast cancer to studies that address quality-of-life issues that affect the patient. Most clinical trials are carried out in phases. Each phase is designed to learn different information, and each builds upon the information previously discovered. Patients may be eligible for studies in different phases, depending on their stage of disease and therapies anticipated, as well as treatment they have already had. Patients are monitored at specific intervals while participating in studies.

> *Phase I studies* are used to find the best way to do a new treatment and how much of it can be given safely. In such studies, only a small number of patients are asked to participate. They are offered to patients whose cancer cannot be helped by other known treatment modalities. Usually, these patients are battling metastatic breast cancer and have exhausted other treatment options. Some patients have personally received benefit from participation, but most have experienced no benefit in fighting their cancer. They are, however, paving the way for the next generation, which is important. Once the optimum dose is chosen, the drug is studied for its ability to shrink tumors in phase II trials.

Phase II studies are designed to discover if the treatment actually kills cancer cells in patients. A slightly larger cohort of patients is selected for this trial, usually between 20 and 50. Patients whose breast cancer has no longer responded to other known treatments may be offered participation in this type of trial. Tumor shrinkage is measured, and patients are closely observed to measure the treatment's effects. If at least 20 percent of patients in this study respond to treatment, the treatment is considered to be successful. Side effects are also closely monitored and carefully recorded and addressed.

Phase III studies usually compare standard treatments already in use with treatments that appeared to be good in small cohort phase II trials. This level requires large numbers of patients to participate, usually thousands. Patients are randomized for the treatment regimen they will be receiving. These studies seek benefits of longer survival, better quality of life, fewer side effects, and fewer cases of cancer recurrence. This is the most common type of clinical trial you may hear about and be asked to participate in.

Adjuvant studies are conducted to determine if additional therapy will further improve the chances for long-term survival and for a reduction of the risk of recurrence. This study progresses through phase I, II, and III trials like other treatment studies.

Supportive care studies are tailored to improve ways of managing side effects caused by treatment. They also include some quality-of-life studies as well.

Prevention studies focus on patients at high risk of developing breast cancer or potentially having a recurrence of disease. These studies commonly will be geared toward one group in the cohort taking a medication or some type of therapy and the other group of the study not receiving anything or receiving a placebo. There are also some studies that focus on early detection and methods of diagnosing breast cancer sooner, even before it becomes actual cancer.

The following is a list of questions that may help guide you in decision making and fact finding about clinical trials associated with high-risk status or breast cancer diagnosis and treatment:

What is the purpose of the study?

How many people will be included in the study?

What does the study involve?

What kind of tests and treatment will I have?

How are treatments given, and what side effects might I expect?

What are the risks and benefits of each protocol?

How long will the study last?

What type of long-term follow-up care is provided for those who participate?

Will I incur any costs? Will my insurance company pay for part of this?

When will the results be known?

Realize that a woman may derive substantial benefit from participating in clinical trials. Every successful cancer treatment being used today started as a clinical trial. Those patients who participated in these studies were the first to benefit. Participation can therefore potentially benefit you. Perhaps equally as important (and to some, more important), you may be contributing in a major way for the next generation dealing with this disease.

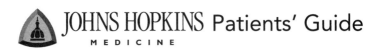

CHAPTER 4

JOHNS HOPKINS Patients' Guide
MEDICINE

Be Prepared—
The Side Effects of
Treatment

A patient may experience various side effects while receiving treatment for breast cancer. Some are easily controlled and some may be more difficult. No two patients are alike, so don't assume if you knew someone with breast cancer that your situation will mirror hers. The following are some of the more common side effects that should be discussed with your oncology team so you know what to expect regarding the status of your disease and the treatments being recommended on your behalf. This list can look overwhelming. It is not intended to alarm you but to provide you with a thorough, comprehensive list of possible issues that may need to be addressed while undergoing treatment.

ANEMIA

Anemia is a common problem for many dealing with cancer. It is especially an issue for those undergoing chemotherapy. By definition, anemia is an abnormally low level of red blood cells (RBCs). These cells contain hemoglobin (an iron protein) that provides oxygen to all parts of the body. If RBC levels are low, one part of the body may not be receiving all the oxygen it needs to work and function well. In general, people with anemia commonly report feeling tired. The fatigue that is associated with anemia can seriously affect quality of life for some patients and make it difficult for patients to cope at times.

Medications such as Procrit (epoetin) or Aranesp (darbepoetin) may be recommended to stimulate your bone marrow to make more red blood cells, thus raising your blood cell count and increasing your energy level. Such a medication is given by injection under the skin using a very small, thin needle. The doses vary, and it is common to be given one of these medications for this side effect once a week. You also might be advised to take an oral iron supplement while receiving these injections.

CARDIAC CHANGES

Several drugs can produce heart problems. Adriamycin (doxorubicin), a chemotherapy agent, and Herceptin, a biological targeted agent, are two such drugs. To help determine if it is safe and appropriate to give someone these medications, an echocardiogram (ECHO) or MUGA (multiple-gated acquisition) scan is done prior to beginning therapy. For women in need of both drugs, an ECHO or

MUGA scan may be done every few months to reevaluate the heart function and ensure that all is well. Upon completion of Herceptin, the scan is repeated again. Congestive heart failure, a weakness of the heart muscle, can occur but is not common. Heart failure also can occur but is rare, mild, and usually treated successfully. The key is close monitoring. Some women are given Herceptin alone with a very low risk to their heart.

COGNITIVE DYSFUNCTION

People receiving chemotherapy as part of their cancer treatment sometimes can have trouble remembering names, places, or events, or they may have trouble concentrating or doing arithmetic. This is referred to as cognitive dysfunction or as some might say, "chemo brain." Currently, this is an area of scientific study that tries to better understand what is causing the dysfunction and how to counteract it. If you are finding that these symptoms are fairly severe and impacting your ability to function well, ask your family to assist you with such things as balancing your checkbook. Make a list of things you need to do and mark each item off as you do it. Keep your keys in the same place so they are easier to find each time you need them. Most importantly, get your family members to assist you with medication management. Rather than relying on your memory, it might be a good idea to use a pill box that has the times of day to take your medications.

After chemotherapy is completed, these symptoms usually subside in time. It's of importance to note that some breast cancer patients who have not had chemotherapy report having these symptoms, too. Therefore, researchers have questioned whether part of the problem with memory and concentration could be related to post-traumatic stress disorder. When individuals experience a traumatic event, the stress can cause residual fears and anxieties. This is a common issue for people in the military who return from war. Remember, you actually are going to "war" with your breast cancer, so it makes sense to some degree that just like a soldier returning from the battlefield, things can feel foggy for a bit.

FATIGUE

Feeling exhausted or extremely tired is probably the most common side effect patients report. This can happen as a side effect of chemotherapy and/or radiation therapy. Fatigue can also be triggered by anemia. If there are specific problems (such as difficulty sleeping) that are related to fatigue, make your doctor aware of them so that she or he might prescribe something to help you sleep better. Also ask about how to better cope with your emotional distress, which can increase fatigue. Conserving your energy is important so that you are spending your time doing things that are important to you. Make a list of the activities and chores you are trying to accomplish—food shopping, work, housecleaning, and the like—and see about recruiting the help of family and friends. You may also notice that your energy level is better during certain times of the day. The Oncology Nursing Society has a website that provides some specific recommendations related to this side effect. Take a look at http://www.cancersymptoms.org/symptoms/fatigue/. Also visit the National Comprehensive Cancer Network's website for more information at http://www.nccn.org.

LYMPHEDEMA

Lymphedema is an abnormal collection of lymph fluid in the arms or legs. Lymphatic fluid is in our bodies to fight infection and cancer. When a relatively large number of lymph nodes have been surgically removed or irradiated, the pathway for lymphatic drainage can become disrupted, and fluid may have trouble returning back up the arm. This results in the arm swelling and staying that way. Infection, trauma to the arm, or other factors may trigger the lymphedema to occur. Lymphedema can cause discomfort and pain, and may limit your arm's use due to the swelling. The incidence of lymphedema is lower in the last 15 years because of improvements in surgical (sentinel node biopsy) and radiation therapy techniques. If you develop lymphedema, you may experience a heavy, throbbing pain or soreness and a feeling of tightness from your wristwatch, rings, or clothing.

Some steps you can take to help prevent lymphedema include the following:

- Perform gentle strengthening and stretching exercises to keep the affected arm working normally.

- Avoid lifting or moving heavy objects with that arm after surgery.

- Keep the skin clean and moisturized, avoid cuts or cracks in the skin, and avoid insect bites whenever possible.

- Avoid needle sticks in that arm; this includes IVs, vaccinations, or blood drawn from the arm where lymph nodes were surgically removed and/or irradiated.

- Avoid having your blood pressure taken in that arm.

- Report signs of infection to your doctor right away. If you do get a cut or injury to this arm, wash the cut immediately and apply an over-the-counter antibiotic ointment right away.

- Report any changes you notice to this arm, such as swelling or feeling of heaviness.

If you develop lymphedema, there are several treatments that may be helpful. These treatments include elevation of the arm, use of a special arm stocking (known as a compression sleeve), massage by a rehabilitation therapist who specializes in lymphedema management, compression bandaging, and a pressure pump. For more information about lymphedema, contact the National Lymphedema Network at 800-541-3259 or visit their website at http://www.lymphnet.org.

HAIR LOSS

The technical term is alopecia, but the term patients recognize most clearly is exactly what it is—hair loss. The hair on your head falls out, and if hair on other parts of your body grows rapidly, it may also fall out (such as eyelashes or eyebrows.) This is a relatively common side effect of several chemotherapy agents used to treat and manage breast cancer. Hair loss in society has become a signal that the person without hair may be a cancer patient. It can be psychologically and physically difficult to cope with hair loss because it is associated with our self-image, womanliness, health status, and other personal issues.

Getting a wig in advance of hair loss can be helpful so that your hair style, texture, and color can be matched well for you. Some insurance companies cover the expense of a wig. Check your policy and see if your insurance company covers "skull prosthesis for side effects of cancer treatment." Costs that are not covered are tax deductible. There are programs like "Look Good, Feel Good" that most cancer centers offer to their patients. This is a special program available free of charge to show you how to wear turbans, scarves, and makeup to reduce the obvious appearance of hair loss. Ask your doctor or nurse when they are offering this program at the facility where you are getting your treatment. If the chemotherapy agents your doctor is recommending are known to cause hair loss, anticipate your hair loss occurring between 10 and 14 days after your first chemotherapy treatment.

Some patients decide to be proactive and take charge of their hair loss themselves rather than waiting for it to happen. Doing your own buzz cut can be therapeutic so that you are determining when your hair departs rather than waiting for the drug to do it.

INFECTION

When harmful bacteria, viruses, or fungi enter the body and the body is not able to destroy these cells by using its immune system, an infection brews. Breast cancer patients are at a higher risk of developing an infection because the cancer present in their body along with the treatments being given can weaken their immune system. Spiking a high fever, chills, sweating, sore throat, mouth sores, pain or burning during urination, diarrhea, shortness of breath, a productive cough, swelling, redness, or pain around an incision or wound are symptoms that an infection may be present.

To help reduce your risk of infection, try to stay away from young children who may be carrying flu viruses, colds, and other respiratory illnesses. Young children can look relatively healthy while harboring germs. This doesn't mean to abandon seeing your children or grandchildren, though. It does mean to evaluate how the child is feeling and if he or she has any symptoms (runny nose, fever, cough) that would signal that this isn't a good day to have the child sitting on your lap. You and family members who live with or frequently see you should receive flu vaccinations to help reduce the risk of unknowingly bringing viruses your way. At the early signs you may be getting an infection (fever, cold, etc.), notify your doctor so he or she can prescribe something for you.

MENOPAUSAL SYMPTOMS

Approximately 40 percent of women dealing with breast cancer develop menopausal symptoms due to breast cancer treatments. This can particularly be an issue for women who are premenopausal and are undergoing chemotherapy and/or hormonal therapy for treatment of their disease. It is thought to be caused by a decline in estrogen and other hormones. These symptoms can include hot flashes, night sweats, vaginal dryness, pain during intercourse, difficulty with bladder control, insomnia, and depression. Some patients take various forms of complementary therapies to try to reduce symptoms. These include vitamins, soy products, black cohosh, and other preparations. Presently, there aren't studies to give definitive answers about the use of these supplements. It is worth talking to your doctor, however, about his or her thoughts regarding various supplements.

Some patients find that taking a medication like Effexor (venlafaxine) can be helpful in reducing hot flashes. There are also some other medications in the same drug category as this one (antidepressants) that may be recommended to help reduce hot flashes. Wearing cotton clothing in layers that can be peeled off as needed also can be helpful. There are various vaginal lubricants that can be used for vaginal dryness and pain during intercourse. These include Replens, Astroglide, or K-Y Jelly. Avoid using petroleum-based products because this can increase your risk of vaginal infections. Avoid spicy foods, smoking, alcohol, caffeine, hot showers, and hot weather, all of which can trigger hot flashes.

MOUTH SORES

Also known as mucositis, a mouth sore is an inflammation of the inside of the mouth and throat, and can result in painful ulcers. Certain medications like steroids may increase the risk of developing an infection in your mouth. Keep your mouth clean and moist to prevent infection. Brush your teeth with a soft-bristled toothbrush after each meal and rinse regularly. Avoid commercial mouthwashes that contain alcohol because they can irritate the mouth. If you wear dentures that are not fitting properly, you will be more likely to get sores in your mouth from rubbing and irritation. This can be a problem particularly if you have experienced or are experiencing weight loss because your gums may shrink, changing the fit of your dentures. See your dentist for evaluation of this. If you have dental needs that have not been taken care of prior to starting chemotherapy, ask your oncologist and dentist to talk on the phone and discuss what strategy to use to reduce risk of infection and mouth sores while receiving your treatments.

NAUSEA AND VOMITING

These are relatively common side effects associated with chemotherapy drugs. However, with the development of newer antinausea medicines (called antiemetics), the incidence of nausea and vomiting has been reduced considerably. Still, when beginning new medications such as hormonal therapy, these side effects may be problematic for a time. Pain medications have a reputation for contributing to nausea too. If it is severe, resulting in an inability to eat or retain foods, dehydration can result. Changes in what you eat and drink may be useful in managing nausea and vomiting. Some specific suggestions include:

Eat a light meal before each chemotherapy treatment.

Eat small amounts of food and liquids at a time.

Eat bland foods and liquids.

Eat dry crackers when feeling nauseated.

Limit the amount of liquids you take with your meals.

Maintain adequate liquids in between meals; drink mostly clear liquids such as water, apple juice, herbal tea, or bouillon.

Eat cool foods or foods at room temperature.

Avoid foods with strong odors.

Avoid high-fat, greasy, and fried foods.

Avoid spicy foods, alcohol, and caffeine.

Suck on peppermint candies as an additional way to help reduce and/or prevent nausea.

Rub peppermint lip balm above your lip and below your nose so that you are smelling mint as a way to reduce nausea.

Ask your oncologist for a prescription for an antiemetic, and ask if you can take it in a preventative manner to prevent, reduce, and control nausea. These medicines include such drugs as Zofran (ondansetron), Kytril (granisetron), Compazine (prochlorperazine), and Emend (aprepitant).

NEUROLOGICAL PROBLEMS

Peripheral neuropathy is a term you might hear as a possible side effect of some chemotherapy drugs. This term describes damage to peripheral nerves. There are three types of peripheral nerves: sensory, motor, and autonomic. Sensory nerves allow us to feel temperature, pain, vibration, and touch. Motor nerves are responsible for voluntary movement and basically allow us to walk and open doors, for example. Autonomic nerves control involuntary or automatic functions such as breathing, digestion of food, and bowel and bladder activities. When there is damage to the peripheral nerves, the symptoms are dependent on the type of peripheral nerves affected. Though chemotherapy drugs can affect any of the peripheral nerves, the most common ones affected are the sensory nerves, causing numbness and tingling in the hands and feet. For patients who already have peripheral neuropathy from other causes (diabetes, for example), chemotherapy can sometimes make it worse. Symptoms of peripheral neuropathy include:

- Numbness and tingling (which may feel like pins and needles in your hands and/or feet)

- Burning pain in your hands and feet

- Difficulty writing or buttoning a shirt

- Difficulty holding a cup or glass

- Constipation

- Decreased sensation of hot or cold

- Muscle weakness

- Decreased hearing or ringing in the ears (known as tinnitus)

If you develop any of these symptoms, it is important to tell your doctor right away. Describe for him or her the symptoms you are experiencing. If you already have any of these symptoms before starting chemotherapy, make your doctor aware of this as well. Your doctor may decide to prescribe medication to reduce these symptoms. The medicines most commonly used are drugs given to neurology patients for treatment of seizures and depression, and may include one or several of the following: Neurontin (gabapentin), Tegretol (carbamazepine), and Elavil (amitriptyline). Some additional measures you should consider taking at home include paying close attention to your walking and removing any scatter rugs from your house. Keep your home well lit so you can see where you are walking. If you are still driving a car, be sure you can actually feel the foot pedals. If temperatures are hard to determine, then ask for help in checking the temperature of the bathtub as well as hot beverages.

SEXUAL DYSFUNCTION

The percentage of women dealing with breast cancer who experience problems continuing sexual activity isn't clearly known. Even for the general population of women not dealing with breast cancer, 43 percent have reported problems having sexual activity for a myriad of reasons. Some patients find it very difficult to comfortably discuss this issue with their doctor, though it may be very important to their quality of life. Side effects from treatment may result in a lower libido; weight gain, fatigue, or other symptoms because of hair loss; and simply not feeling well enough to try or confident enough to engage in sexual activity. Physical intimacy is one aspect of a loving relationship. It gives us personal pleasure and creates a feeling of closeness to our partner. Sexual intercourse, however, is just one way of being physically intimate. Cuddling, hugging, touching, rubbing, and holding hands are all pleasurable ways to show one another affection. Talking with your partner about your concerns and feelings will allow you to help one another. Experiment with different positions too; you may find that one may be more comfortable than another when having sex. Vaginal lubricants also can help with vaginal dryness. Some women who have not had success with commercial vaginal lubricants have tried egg whites for lubrication. (Be sure to wash thoroughly after intercourse. Do not use douche solutions, however.) If a lack of energy impairs sexual activity, plan ahead for intimacy by identifying when you are feeling higher levels of energy during certain times of the day or week. Vaginal discharge, burning, or itching may be signs of a vaginal infection. See your gynecologist if you develop these symptoms so they can be properly treated.

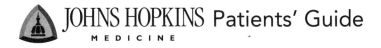

CHAPTER 5

JOHNS HOPKINS Patients' Guide

M E D I C I N E

STRAIGHT TALK—
COMMUNICATION WITH
FAMILY, FRIENDS, AND
COWORKERS

The feelings of shock, concern, and confusion you felt when you were diagnosed with cancer will also be experienced by friends and loved ones when they hear the news. Who you will tell and when you will tell them will vary, depending on their relationship to you and how they will be impacted. Family members, others who live with you, your boss, and close friends will be aware that you are experiencing great stress. Your treatment is likely to change their routines as well as your own and to have an emotional impact on them, too.

TALKING TO YOUNG CHILDREN

How and when to tell a child his or her mother has cancer is a difficult decision, no matter what the age of the child. Undoubtedly your children will realize that something difficult is going on. It is best to be honest with your children, because they are likely to overhear conversations, even if you do not talk to them directly. Keeping the truth from your children will likely make them more scared than comforted. Depending on your family, it may make sense for either one or both parents to talk with the children. Explain to them in clear terms how treatment will get rid of the cancer. Many parents choose to wait to tell their children until after they've seen the doctors and know the treatment plans. It is important to remember that some treatments for breast cancer may alter your physical appearance (like hair loss), and it is important to prepare your children or grandchildren for that possibility.

Depending on the age and maturity level of the child, it may be worth considering attending a support group for patients with breast cancer during your treatment. In addition, many major cancer centers will offer educational programs for children to introduce them to the hospital and treatments to help reduce their fears and anxieties regarding the unknown. If your children have many questions about your treatment, attending such a program with them may help to reduce their fears and uncertainty.

Toddlers and preschoolers are very dependent on their parents and, as a result, are quick to notice stress or tension in the home. Don't assume that their age prevents them from feeling your stress. Though children of this age won't understand what cancer is, you can let them know that you are very sick and that the doctors are going to work very hard to make you better. Your young children may be worried that you will go away like other relatives who have passed on. Though you may not be able to assure them this will not happen to you, acknowledging their fears may be critical to their well-being. They may also feel as though something they did caused you to be ill. It is important to reassure children that your illness is not their fault. It is also a good idea to tell your children that sometimes you will feel sad or tired and that this is also not their fault. Let them know it is okay for them to be sad and that they can talk to you or your partner any time they are feeling sad. Try to maintain family routines as much as possible.

TALKING WITH SCHOOL-AGE CHILDREN AND TEENS

If your children are older, they may be anxious or even angry about how this will impact them. Teens often view the world as revolving around them, and they may resent how changes in routine will impact them. These natural teen responses can be magnified by their fear of losing a parent. Because every child is different, it is important to know where they are coming from mentally and emotionally. Keeping communication lines open is critical, particularly for children in this age group. You will have to decide who will tell the kids and when, but also how much detail you want to share with them and at what intervals. Their knowledge of cancer in general may be to associate it with death. Ask your son or daughter what they know about cancer and then provide them with details at their level. Reassure them honestly about your treatment and prognosis.

Teens may be particularly resentful when asked to help out around the house. There is some evidence that teens are unable to psychologically cope with the responsibility of filling a parent's role during such times of upheaval. Teens may then feel guilty about their feelings of resentment, further compounding an unfortunate situation. Discover ways for the older child to contribute to the family while maintaining typical roles and boundaries as much as possible. Explain to them that you may need extra help around the house for a while, but also take steps to show balance between family responsibilities and normal teenage lifestyles. Discuss how the family will work to balance responsibilities.

TELLING OTHER FAMILY MEMBERS

Telling other family members can also be difficult. Mothers in particular are used to making everything better for their children and may want to try to control the situation for you. They may be frustrated when they can't guide or control your treatment and recovery. They will need to be given constructive ways to help because no matter what, they will want to help you—even if you feel you don't need it. Mothers can fill an important role in the home if there are children to care for.

Other family members will also have unique relationships that need to be considered. Siblings may also feel great grief and concern for your well-being. Having them assist with information gathering can help engage them in your treatment and empower them with education that will help both of you. Family can also be critical for providing and coordinating assistance during your treatment. Remember that every offer for assistance is genuine, and be ready to accept assistance. Keep your family members informed of how you are doing as treatment progresses. Remember, this is a disease that affects the entire family. The feelings of fear and apprehension you have are shared by many.

WHAT TO TELL YOUR BOSS AND COWORKERS

Whether to inform coworkers about your illness is a very personal decision. There are advantages to letting key people know because you will more than likely require some time off for treatment. You may choose to tell only your supervisor or your closest associates, or you may decide to be very public about your situation.

It is common to be concerned about maintaining your job after treatment. Fortunately, the American Disabilities Act (ADA) provides some job protection. You should be able to work with your boss on a schedule that will meet your medical needs as well as the needs of your employer. You are not actually required to tell your supervisor you have cancer. It is fine to explain that you are under doctor's care that will require you to miss time from work. Most individuals, however, will tell their boss that they have been diagnosed with cancer and will be undergoing whatever treatments have been recommended. You are not responsible for providing information about your prognosis.

As with friends and family, deciding what to tell coworkers can be difficult. Many people will choose to inform coworkers in vague terms rather than to provide the full details of their treatment plan. Again, this is your personal business, and whatever feels right in your situation is the best answer. As with family, offers of assistance from friends and coworkers are typically genuine, and it is beneficial for you as well as the helpers to involve them as needed.

KEEPING FRIENDS AND FAMILY UPDATED

During and after treatment, the need to update people on your situation can be a job in and of itself. You may want to assign someone to be the "information center" to provide all announcements about how you are doing, what treatment you are having, pathology results, and so on. There are also a number of online resources for posting such information that are usually free, can be personalized, and serve as your website to keep friends and family informed during difficult times. Some websites include a patient care journal to update family and friends, a photo gallery, and a guest book where visitors can post messages of support and encouragement. Email is another good way to make sure that everyone is receiving the most current information at the same time and in the same manner. Have one of your family or friends who want to help gather important email addresses, and enlist someone to send out broadcast emails to everyone at once. You will find such options to be a great time saver to help reduce the burden on you and to ensure consistency in the information being provided. It also helps prevent hurt feelings if one person finds out you called someone else first.

HOW TO RECRUIT SUPPORT FROM FAMILY AND FRIENDS

People will undoubtedly ask what they can do to help you. It may be helpful to identify a coordinator early on who can delegate tasks to your support team. Among the many things people can do are help drive you to appointments, drive your children to school and events, run errands, make meals (that can be put in the freezer), babysit, help with the housework, or add you to prayer lists at church. Remember that these people want to do something to help and would not offer if they did not sincerely want to provide assistance. One day, you will be able to reciprocate perhaps and help them in a crisis.

On the other hand, some friends may avoid calling you after they hear the news. It isn't that they don't care; it's more likely that they don't know what to say. Let them know that even though the diagnosis is upsetting to hear, you need their support. Remember that support from others is an important part of your treatment plan for you and your family.

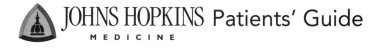

CHAPTER 6

JOHNS HOPKINS Patients' Guide
M E D I C I N E

MAINTAINING BALANCE— WORK AND LIFE DURING TREATMENT

HOW TO PLAN CARE AND MINIMIZE DISRUPTIONS IN YOUR LIFE

Women are used to being the caregiver, not the one needing care. Women are accustomed to juggling busy schedules and functioning as wife, mother, nurse, babysitter, financial manager, counselor, chauffeur, and magician in the family most of the time. For this reason, women sometimes aren't good at asking for and accepting help from others. Breast cancer treatment will alter roles, play havoc with schedules, and create additional stress for the patient, other family members, and friends helping during this time. Disruptions are inevitable, but very manageable.

PREPARING CHILDREN FOR YOUR TREATMENTS

Patients with children especially may experience a variety of role changes. Daddy may be putting young children to bed because Mommy doesn't feel well tonight. Older children may be asked to help with meal preparation or laundry. It's important for you and your family to talk about your schedules and how treatment needs will impact them, and to design a new schedule to best meet your needs and those of your loved ones—with as little change as possible.

This is also the time to ask for and accept help from other family members, neighbors, and friends in caring for your kids. After all, one day they may need your help in a very similar way.

Try to maintain your children's routines as much as possible. Change creates stress no matter what the age—even an infant who is fed an hour later than usual expresses his opinions about his altered schedule. Let your children know in advance if there will be a change in their routine.

Keep children informed about what is happening related to treatment. Encourage them to help and play an active role in the treatment, too. Have elementary school-aged children (ages 6–12) go with you to the hospital when you get one of your chemotherapy treatments to better understand what is happening. Ask them how they picture the chemotherapy traveling through your veins destroying any bad cells that might be lingering somewhere. Have them draw pictures to cheer you up. They can open the get-well cards you receive in the mail too. Explain why you don't feel well and the importance of playing quietly on certain days after treatment. Let young children know they can't catch breast cancer and also aren't in any way the cause of it.

PREPARING FOR SURGERY

In preparation for surgery, request to meet with a breast center nurse for some preoperative consultation. You will want to know in advance if you will be having any drains in place, how long you will be out of commission from doing your routine activities, what clothing will be best to wear postoperatively, when you will be allowed to resume driving, and so forth. Most women today are good candidates for lumpectomy with sentinel node biopsy. If you fall into this category for surgical treatment, anticipate a fairly short time of being unable to do your routine. No drains are required. You can resume driving the next morning and can technically even go back to work as long as it doesn't involve heavy lifting. For women having mastectomy without reconstruction, recovery is about 2–3 weeks and one drain is in place. For women having mastectomy with some form of reconstruction, recovery is longer and dependent on the type of reconstruction done. (Three weeks for women having mastectomy with tissue expander, and 5–6 weeks for those having mastectomy with flap reconstruction.) This is why it's good to formally meet with a breast center nurse to learn about what to expect, when, and for how long. You may have several drains in this case.

PREPARING FOR CHEMOTHERAPY

If you are scheduled to have chemotherapy, make a chart of when your treatments will be. See about having chemotherapy appointments toward the end of the week so you can have the weekend to rest up (when hopefully there will be additional help around the house available to you). Decide if you want someone to go with you for chemotherapy treatments. You will be in the chemotherapy infusion center for several hours, so plan accordingly. The day needs to be as laid back as possible for you. Depending on who is available to help and what the schedule is, you may decide the chemotherapy days are "pizza night" for the kids or time to reheat that casserole your neighbor made.

In anticipation of hair loss, consider being proactive and getting your hair cut short or even doing your own buzz cut prior to your hair falling out. A "coming-out party" for your hair, as mentioned earlier, can be fun to do and is a good way to engage your teens and preteens in your upcoming treatment.

PREPARING FOR RADIATION

For radiation, consider scheduling it at the very beginning or the end of the day rather than in the middle. Since this treatment is daily, you will want it to cause as little disruption to your daily routine as possible. Most radiation facilities have patients in and out in under 30 minutes. You spend more time getting your clothes on and off than you do actually receiving your treatment.

CONTINUING WORK

Most women continue to work while receiving their breast cancer treatment. Time missed from work is usually minimal, if planned relatively well. It is actually to your advantage to continue to work because stopping work can be an additional stressor for you; it changes your routine abruptly. You want to continue to feel productive, be surrounded by supportive coworkers, and not be spending every waking moment thinking about cancer. Sit down with your supervisor and plan a schedule that works for both of you. There may be some days you work only half a day because you are getting chemotherapy in the afternoon, then taking off the following day. During radiation, you may be coming in an hour later to work or leaving 30 minutes early to get to your daily radiation appointment. Bosses know the importance of being flexible, and you are protected to some degree by the family medical leave act. If you work around small children though, especially the toddler age, this may be problematic during chemotherapy because your risk of getting an infection is increased during this time.

WHEN YOU MIGHT EXPECT NOT TO FEEL WELL

Being prepared for side effects helps you plan your schedule day to day and week to week as well as gives you a better sense of control during a time of stress and change. For women having chemotherapy, usually if you are going to have GI (gastrointestinal) side effects, they will be 16–48 hours after the infusion of the chemotherapy drugs was completed. How you tolerate the first chemotherapy sets the stage for how other sessions using the same medicines will go. Request antinausea medications in advance so you can also head off any GI symptoms prior to their occurrence.

For women receiving radiation as part of their treatment, anticipate feeling fine until about the last 2 weeks or so of radiation. At this point, you may notice increased fatigue. This is because radiation is accumulative. Give yourself extra time to rest at night and even take a catnap in the middle of the day, if possible.

INFECTION PREVENTION TO STAY HEALTHY DURING TREATMENT

During chemotherapy, there will be certain days that it will be anticipated that your white blood cells will go down in response to having received chemotherapy. These are days you are more vulnerable to getting a cold, flu, or other form of infection. You want to avoid being in the presence of young children because they can be sick even without appearing so. Wearing a mask is beneficial if you can't avoid being around them in a closed environment.

Eating a balanced diet, rich in fruits and vegetables, helps to improve your immune system. Washing your hands frequently is smart, too. Getting a flu shot before you start chemotherapy is advisable as well. Have your teeth cleaned and any dental work that needs to be done before you start chemotherapy to prevent any later problems related to tooth infections. (Chemotherapy doesn't cause dental problems, but if a tooth infection is brewing, it can be made worse due to your immune system being taxed and unable to fight infection as well as it did before.) If you need to travel by air while undergoing chemotherapy, wear a mask to reduce your risk of exposure. If it is winter, be sure to bundle up when outdoors. Your mission is to be healthy during your chemotherapy treatments and to reduce the risk of exposure to infection as much as possible. The nurse working with you during your chemotherapy treatments can mark on your chart the days that you will be particularly vulnerable to infection. Your blood will be periodically drawn to assess how your body's immune system is responding to the treatments and whether any medicines to boost your white blood cells need to be given.

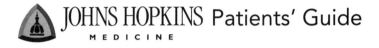

CHAPTER 7

JOHNS HOPKINS Patients' Guide
MEDICINE

Surviving Breast Cancer— Reengaging in Mind and Body Health After Treatment

SURVIVORSHIP

When do you consider yourself a survivor? The most common definition is actually the moment you are diagnosed and have chosen to embark on treatment. Some people, however, don't consider themselves survivors until treatment is completed (with perhaps the exception of still being on hormonal therapy). There are millions of women (and several thousand men) who are breast cancer survivors. You are among an elite group. When you finish your treatment, however, rather than feeling like celebrating, you may feel like you fell off a cliff. This is not an unusual reaction either. You've been so focused on actively fighting this disease that when it is time to stop, you feel a sense of letdown—fear, too, that you haven't done enough, or that there isn't an additional treatment to prevent recurrence. Fear of recurrence remains the biggest concern for survivors. Though the majority of women won't ever face recurrence of this disease, it can be hard to learn to trust your body again. Staying in the know about the latest research that has been published about breast cancer is helpful and empowering. Taking measures to help yourself regain emotional balance is wise too. Some breast centers offer special survivor retreats for this purpose.

COUNSELING

If your doctor or nurse recommends that you consider seeing a counselor, don't feel like you have failed at getting yourself back on track. It's hard. Many women would benefit from seeing a therapist posttreatment to help them reengage in their lives physically and emotionally. Sometimes you simply need a professional sounding board to hear your hidden thoughts and fears and to help you gain perspective about what to (and what not to) worry about. You want to regain control over your life. Doing so might require assistance from others who are professionally trained at doing this. Diagnosis and treatment of breast cancer is a life-altering experience. There is no operator's manual for this experience. Talk with other survivors, too, to help you realize that what you are experiencing is the norm and not the exception.

MANAGING LONG-TERM SIDE EFFECTS OF TREATMENT

It would be great if at the time treatment ended, all the side effects associated with it ended too, but this is not the case. You may be dealing with residual side effects of bone/joint pain, peripheral neuropathy, difficulty concentrating, fatigue, hot flashes, night sweats, or other unpleasantness. Give your body time to heal and adjust. Some side effects like fatigue can linger for a year. If you are taking hormonal therapy, you may experience menopausal symptoms until this adjuvant therapy is completed. You may still be doing some final touch-ups on your reconstruction too, which require additional surgery. Don't expect to feel back to yourself the week treatments end. There is a period of psychological and physical adjustment, similar to becoming pregnant and 9 months later giving birth. Your body needs time. Allow it this time. (See Chapter 4 for management of side effects.)

LIVING A HEALTHIER LIFESTYLE

Taking charge of your health and psychological well-being should be a priority for you now. The following are some helpful ways to accomplish this and feel good doing it.

NUTRITION

If you eat healthier and watch your weight, you may help to reduce your risk of this disease recurring. Experts know that high-fat diets that encourage packing on the pounds can increase risk due to the additional weight gain (which translates into more estrogen being stored in body fat).

Eating a diet rich in green and orange vegetables is smart for your breast health as well as your heart. This doesn't mean that you have to give up chocolate nut sundaes for the rest of your life. Eat smart. Save high-fat and high-calorie foods for special times; just don't make them part of your daily life.

If you are currently overweight, consider joining a group to help you reduce weight gradually. Avoid diet pills and fad diets. Changing eating habits and making it part of your lifestyle is what will take the weight off and keep it off. It needs to be an overall program and not something temporary. Women usually have better success at losing weight when they partner with someone else who shares the same goal. Heart-healthy menus are also breast-healthy menus.

EXERCISE

This is another way to help reduce the risk of recurrence. This doesn't mean you need to become a marathon runner and press 400 pounds at the gym. It does mean finding an exercise program that works for you, that you can commit to, and makes you feel good. If you enjoy the exercise program, if it is in an environment that makes you feel comfortable, if you feel better after you do it, and if it is something you are able to stick with, then it's a winner for you. Power walking is a good option. Walking three times a week for an hour will suffice. Working out three times a week also will. Again, exercising with a friend usually makes it more enjoyable and helps you to stick to it because you will have a buddy rooting you on.

STRESS

Emotional turmoil affects your immune system, and your immune system needs to be in good shape to fight cancer cells and prevent cancer cells from growing. Though it's a nice fantasy to picture yourself worry free, sitting on a beach nibbling on bonbons, this isn't reality. You will be expected to resume your chaotic life, including family responsibilities and work duties. Reassessing how you react to stressful situations is something you can do, however. Breast cancer can teach you that you really don't have to sweat the small stuff. Making time for you is important, including after treatment is completed. Put things into perspective before reacting to them. Is it really a crisis that your mother-in-law came over and you haven't dusted or vacuumed? You've been through much bigger and more significant stuff. Learn deep-breathing techniques, take a yoga class, or do other forms of relaxation therapy. These can be helpful in reducing stress and keeping life in perspective.

SMOKE AND ALCOHOL

Avoid smoke—and this includes secondary smoke. The American Cancer Society has reported that if all tobacco products no longer existed, 80% of cancers in general would disappear and no longer be a health risk. If you have a friend who smokes, remind her that if she cares about you, she will take her cigarettes outside. If she refuses and still smokes around you, then she isn't your friend. Drinking excessive amounts of alcohol may cause cancer. It doesn't mean you need to give up social drinking, but you should limit alcohol to only one drink a day.

A NEW LEASE ON LIFE

You have just completed treatment that was life altering. You have perhaps stared death in the face and survived what you thought wasn't possible to overcome. This is an ideal time to step back and reassess your life, looking at how you want to leave your mark on this earth, now realizing you are going to be around to make that mark. Some women decide they want to go back to school. Others decide they want to spend more time with their families and work part-time rather than full-time. A few even have decided to get a "husbandectomy" after their lumpectomy. It's your call. It's your life.

Consider setting short-term and long-term goals. Some goals may be directed at living a healthier lifestyle; others may be focused on how you want to make a difference for others who follow you and are diagnosed with this disease. You are connected to an extraordinary group of women who share common thoughts, dreams, and fears. Band together to make a difference or strike out on your own regarding how you want to spend the rest of your life. What you thought was important before may have little meaning now. This can be quite confusing, though, to those around you who were expecting things to return to "normal." You need to find your "new normal" and let your family and friends know that you are working hard to accomplish this. This experience has changed you, hopefully for the better, and your life will be considered more precious and valued than it was before. No doubt about it, you have gotten in touch with your own mortality. Communicate your thoughts with your family and friends. Keep a journal to record them. Journaling can be very therapeutic.

SEEING THE WORLD THROUGH DIFFERENT EYES

It can be hard for people you spend time with—family, friends, and coworkers—to understand that you aren't the same person you were before your diagnosis. Hopefully, you are different in all the right ways: mindful of how precious life is; never taking anything for granted; and valuing relationships differently perhaps than you did before.

Consider getting involved as a volunteer. One of the best ways to move forward with your experience with breast cancer is to help those who are diagnosed after you. By helping someone else, you help yourself psychologically because although the physical recovery from breast cancer may take a finite time, emotional recovery can take a lifetime. It is usually life altering in a positive way. Consider volunteering where you received your treatments or for a breast cancer organization that has a chapter in your area. This is very rewarding and is a great way to give back, as well as help others and yourself. Educate others and help promote breast cancer awareness in your local community. You can save other women's lives (and breasts) by promoting mammography, breast self-exams, and clinical breast exams. If all women in the United States over the age of 40 got an annual mammogram, the number of deaths from breast cancer each year would be reduced by one-third—that's 15,000 lives a year.

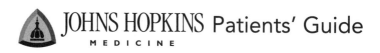

CHAPTER 8

JOHNS HOPKINS Patients' Guide

MEDICINE

MANAGING RISK—
WHAT IF MY CANCER COMES
BACK?

The risk of recurrence remains the most feared issue women deal with when they have finished their treatment. Learning what to look for, when, how, and for how long is helpful. Putting the risk of recurrence into perspective is extremely important to your psychological well-being. For example, if you did a lumpectomy with radiation and now find yourself doing a breast self-exam in the shower every morning, then you aren't enjoying your breast that was purposefully saved.

PREVENTION AND MONITORING FOR RECURRENCE

For women who have undergone lumpectomy and radiation, in general, the risk of recurrence locally in the breast is about 10 percent, perhaps higher for some. How wide the surgical margins were from your breast cancer surgery, what the hormone receptors were, and a few other prognostic factors may influence this number a bit. However, in general, the risk of local recurrence is relatively low, particularly for women diagnosed with early stage breast cancer. Risk of local recurrence is greatest during the first 2 years. Once this milestone is reached, the risk of local recurrence lessens considerably, although it never becomes zero. For women who have had a mastectomy, the risk of local recurrence isn't zero either. It's impossible to remove every bit of breast tissue.

Doing a breast self-exam monthly is important. Now that you have had breast surgery and other treatments, you will need to re-learn what your normal lumps and bumps are. An irradiated breast can go through breast changes for a year after radiation has been completed. It may get firmer, shrink some, or even enlarge some. For women who have had mastectomy without reconstruction, it is still important to check the skin area where the breast once was and look for tiny bumps, especially along the incision line. They may signal a need for further evaluation by your doctor. Women who have had breast reconstruction should continue checking themselves each month too, performing a breast self-exam on their rebuilt breast(s).

If you have undergone a lumpectomy, the surgeon will probably recommend getting mammograms done on that side every 6 months for 2 years, then annually thereafter. For women who have had mastectomy with reconstruction, usually breast imaging studies are not recommended.

If you had cancer in several of your lymph nodes or had a very large tumor ("locally advanced" or stage III), then you probably had some scans done as part of your original staging workup. It no longer is routine to do scans each year. Blood tests in the form of tumor markers also may not be routinely done. Instead, doctors rely on the patient reporting symptoms that may imply there is something going on within a distant organ site. A symptom such as constant low back pain that doesn't go away after several weeks, a chronic cough, weight loss, or other signs may signal that cancer has returned to a distant location. This is known as distant recurrence and is classified as metastatic breast cancer. Certainly this outcome is the greatest worry for survivors. In such cases, the mission of treatment is control of the disease because a cure is not a realistic goal (see Chapter 9).

As you might expect, the risk of recurrence is higher for someone who had a higher stage of cancer than someone with an early stage. Survivors with favorable prognostic factors (such as no cancer in the lymph nodes, and having a hormone receptor positive tumor and HER2neu negative receptors) have a lower incidence of local and/or distant recurrence than someone with unfavorable prognostic factors who was considered to have locally-advanced disease upon initial diagnosis.

TREATMENT OPTIONS (LOCAL VERSUS DISTANT RECURRENCE)

If cancer returns in the breast following lumpectomy with radiation, then the standard of care is surgical. Radiation cannot be repeated on the breast, and a mastectomy must be done. If additional chemotherapy is needed, the drug choices will be different than those that were originally given to you. Cancer that recurs within the breast needs to be evaluated to determine if it is true recurrence (return of the original breast cancer that was there) or if it is a new primary with different prognostic factors. When cancer recurs locally in the breast, most of the time it recurs where it started or very close to the original tumor location.

Ways to reduce risk of recurrence include making some wise lifestyle changes (see Chapter 7) and also, for those taking hormonal therapy, being sure to take it as prescribed. Adherence can be an issue for some women due to side effects. Rather than altering a dosage yourself or stopping therapy altogether, inform your doctor of side effects so he or she can help you overcome them. Hormonal therapy for those who are hormone receptor positive can reduce risk of recurrence by as much as 50 percent; a number worth achieving by taking the therapy as prescribed.

DISTANT RECURRENCE

When breast cancer recurs in a distant organ, the most common sites are the bones, liver, lungs, and brain. This wouldn't be considered liver cancer or lung cancer or bone cancer, but breast cancer cells that have traveled to these organ sites and established themselves there. If the tumor is hormone receptor positive, it's not unusual for the doctor to first use hormonal therapy, rather than chemotherapy, to see if this will get the disease under control (see Chapter 9). Radiation may be used to treat distant disease as well as targeted therapies and other drugs. Chemotherapy also will be considered, depending on the location of the cancer, its prognostic factors, and the patient's general health and age. In some cases, targeted therapy is recommended for women whose tumors are HER2neu positive. This includes treatment of brain metastasis since the drug Tykerb crosses the blood-brain barrier.

Local recurrence of breast cancer has not proven to increase mortality. This is why lumpectomy with radiation is equal from a survival perspective to mastectomy, even if the disease locally recurs. Distant recurrence is the bigger worry, because the disease moving to a distant organ is life threatening.

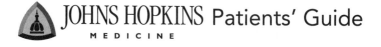

CHAPTER 9

JOHNS HOPKINS Patients' Guide
MEDICINE

MY CANCER ISN'T CURABLE— WHAT NOW?

UNDERSTANDING GOALS OF TREATMENT FOR METASTATIC DISEASE

It can be devastating to hear that your disease has gone beyond the breast and lymphatic system and has been found in another organ. This changes the treatment plan considerably from one of cure to one of control. The mission is controlling the disease and having your body live in harmony with it as long as possible, while maintaining good quality of life. This effort requires a careful balance and can explain why a more conservative-appearing treatment in the form of hormonal therapy or targeted therapy is recommended when you may have anticipated aggressive chemotherapy. The doctors want to see if they can get your body to live in harmony with this disease. It will now be treated like a chronic condition. Consider diabetes, for example; diabetes is a chronic disease that requires ongoing management. If a diabetic didn't take her insulin several times a day, in a matter of a few weeks, she probably would be dead. The same rationale applies for the treatment and control of metastatic breast cancer.

SETTING SHORT-TERM GOALS

Although it would be wonderful to make plans for 10 years from now and expect to be here to carry them out, that may not be realistic. Begin by setting short-term goals. Short-term goals may be 1 year in length. Are there women who have lived a decade or more with metastatic disease? Yes, but unfortunately they are in the minority (though your mission is to be in that minority). Discuss with your doctor what to expect. Be smart; be optimistic but realistic. Don't purchase nonrefundable cruise line tickets for 3 years from now in your name. The goal may be for you to be here in 3 years, but first see how your body responds to treatment of the metastasis before making any assumptions. Ask the doctor how long you will be taking treatment before scans will be repeated to determine the medications' effectiveness in shrinking the cancer.

QUALITY OF LIFE VERSUS QUANTITY OF LIFE

The mission for anyone should be to maintain a good quality of life and to not just focus on how many days, weeks, or years there are left. Quantity of life needs to take a backseat to quality of life. Living a long time in severe pain, unable to take care of your daily needs, and not enjoying still being alive is no way to live. A shorter length of time during which you feel pretty good and are enjoying family is far better than being miserable for a longer length of time. If you are experiencing a great deal of pain, speak up. There are medications to control pain. The doctors and nurses may not know you are suffering if you don't tell them. Sometimes patients are frightened about reporting new symptoms, fearing they will hear that the prognosis is worse. There are situations in which giving a little bit of radiation to the spine, for example, may totally take away back pain. This can only happen by telling the doctor your symptoms and how you feel.

WHEN SHOULD I STOP TREATMENT?

This is not an easy question to ask your doctor and not an easy question for him or her to answer either. Having a candid discussion about this is very valuable—but it may require you to meet with your doctor one-on-one when family isn't accompanying you. It is often easier to talk frankly without your spouse, son, or mother sitting beside you because they don't want to hear the answer to this question. Treatment in general continues as long as you are responding to treatment, there are treatment options to offer you, and your quality of life is being maintained. There is no sense in doing treatment if it isn't helping. You want your doctor to be very honest and open with you. It will be just as hard for him or her to recommend stopping treatment as it will be for you to hear those words. Physicians are trained to make patients better, to heal, to cure, to take pain away, and to reduce suffering. Having to tell someone that continuing treatment isn't going to help accomplish any of these goals is hard, but it is important to state if and when such a time comes.

Being prepared for such a time is wise. This means asking the doctor how long she or he anticipates being able to hold the disease at bay, what drugs in what order you can anticipate being offered and for how long, and the like. Be sure to have your affairs in order and your wishes known. There is a tendency to postpone doing this, perhaps because of denial. Everyone, no matter whether they have cancer or not, should have his or her affairs in order. Life is unpredictable. Fatal car accidents happen, for example. Your situation provides you a window into your future and what timeline it holds for you. Take advantage of this unusual knowledge and make sure you have a will, an advanced directive, your finances in order, and your wishes clearly known to your next of kin.

HOSPICE/PALLIATIVE CARE

When someone reaches the end of his or her life, there are special medical services available to help in preparing to leave this world, including dying with dignity as well as with pain in control, and having your family's emotional needs met. Hospice is an organization that helps make this possible. A referral from your doctor is needed and commonly is arranged around the time the decision is made that treatment is no longer benefitting you. Hospice care can be provided in a hospice facility, in your home, or in the home of a relative. It's your choice. Again, quality of life is paramount. Honoring your wishes and spending time as you want to spend it is the mission now. Counseling is provided to family members, and spiritual needs are addressed for everyone. This is your time with family and friends; this is your time for reflection and to gain a sense of peace. (See the Further Reading section for a book called *100 Questions and Answers About Advanced and Metastatic Breast Cancer.*)

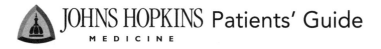

CHAPTER 10

JOHNS HOPKINS Patients' Guide

MEDICINE

BREAST CANCER
IN OLDER ADULTS

By Gary Shapiro, MD

B reast cancer is the most common cancer in women. Contrary to what most people believe, more older women develop and die from breast cancer than do younger women. Breast cancer is a disease of aging. As we live longer, the number of women with breast cancer will increase dramatically. In the next 25 years, the number of people 65 years of age and older will double. The largest increase in cancer incidence will occur in those over 80 years of age.

Older adults with cancer often have other chronic health problems and may be taking multiple medications that can affect their cancer treatment plan. Prejudice, misunder-standing, and limited access to clinical trials often prevent older patients from receiving the timely cancer treatment they need.

Older women may not have adequate screening for breast cancer, and when a cancer is found, it is too often ignored or undertreated. As a result, older women often have worse outcomes than do younger patients. Older women have less breast-conserving surgery, less axillary node sampling, less radiation therapy, and less adjuvant (preventative) chemotherapy. They do not always get appropriate adjuvant hormonal therapy, and their metastatic breast cancer is often left untreated.

WHY IS THERE MORE CANCER IN OLDER PEOPLE?

The organs in our body are made up of cells. Cells divide and multiply according to the needs of the body. Cancer develops when the cells in a specific part of the body grow out of control. The body has a number of ways of repairing damaged control mechanisms, but as we age, these do not work as well. Although our healthier lifestyles have allowed us to avoid death from infection, heart attack, and stroke, we may now live long enough for a cancer to develop. People who live longer have increased exposure to cancer-causing agents (carcinogens) in the environment. Aging decreases the body's ability to protect us from these carcinogens and to repair cells that are damaged by these and other processes.

BREAST CANCER IS DIFFERENT IN OLDER WOMEN

The biology of breast cancer is different in older women than in younger women. As women age, their breast tumors more frequently express hormone receptors, have slower rates of tumor cell growth, and lower overexpression of the HER2neu oncogene. (See Chapters 1 and 3 for more on the biology of breast cancer.) The prognosis for patients with localized and regional stages of breast cancer having these characteristics is usually good. On the other hand, older women with metastases may have a more aggressive disease than do their younger counterparts.

DECISION MAKING: 7 PRACTICAL STEPS

1. GET A DIAGNOSIS

No matter how "typical" the signs and symptoms, first impressions may be wrong. Although most breast masses in older women are malignant, some are benign, or one of the less common "favorable types" of breast cancer that grow to be quite large without metastasizing (for example, mucinous carcinoma). A diagnosis helps you and your family understand what to expect and how to prepare for the future, even if you are not a candidate for curative treatment. Knowing the diagnosis also helps your doctor treat your symptoms. Many people find "not knowing" very hard and are relieved when they finally have an explanation for their symptoms. Sometimes, however, when a frail patient is obviously dying, diagnostic studies can be an additional burden. In such cases, it may be quite reasonable to focus on symptom relief (palliation) without knowing the details of the diagnosis.

2. KNOW THE CANCER'S STAGE

How far the cancer has spread (its stage) defines your prognosis and treatment options. No one can make informed decisions without knowing this. Just as there may be times when the burdens of diagnostic studies may be too great, it may also be appropriate to do without the full battery of staging tests in very frail, dying patients.

As with younger patients, stage is determined by the size of the tumor, the presence or absence of cancer in axillary lymph nodes, or its spread (metastasis) to other organs. When doctors combine this information with information regarding your cancer's hormone receptor and HER2neu status, they can predict what impact, if any, your breast cancer is likely to have on your life expectancy and quality of life.

Approximately 75% of older women with breast cancer have positive estrogen receptors. Though the cancer's stage is still its most important feature, your prognosis is usually better if your cancer is estrogen or progesterone receptor positive. Unfortunately, even early stage, hormone receptor positive breast cancers can recur. Their pattern of recurrence is quite different from that of estrogen receptor negative breast cancers, which have a high risk of early relapse within the first few years. Understanding these distinct timelines is very useful in helping you and your doctor make decisions regarding the benefits of adjuvant hormonal therapy and chemotherapy.

3. KNOW YOUR LIFE EXPECTANCY

Anticancer treatment should be considered if you are likely to live long enough to experience symptoms or premature death from breast cancer. If your life expectancy is so short that the cancer will not significantly affect it, there may be no reason to treat your cancer.

Chronological age (how old you are) should not be the deciding factor of how your cancer should, or should not, be treated. Despite advanced age, women who are relatively well often have a life expectancy that is longer than their life expectancy with breast cancer. The average 70-year-old woman is likely to live another 16 years. A similar 85-year-old can expect to live an additional 6 years and remain independent for most of that time. Even an unhealthy 75-year-old woman can live 5 more years; long enough to suffer symptoms and early death from metastatic breast cancer.

4. UNDERSTAND THE GOALS

The Goals of Treatment

It is important to be clear whether the goal of treatment is cure (adjuvant therapy for early stage breast cancer) or palliation (treatment for incurable advanced metastatic breast cancer). If the goal is palliation, ask if the treatment plan will extend life, control symptoms, or both. How likely is the treatment to achieve these goals, and how long will you enjoy its benefits?

When the goal of treatment is palliation, chemotherapy should never be administered without defined endpoints and timelines. It should be clear to everyone what "counts" as success, how it will be determined (for example, a symptom controlled or a smaller mass on CAT scan), and when. You and your family should understand what your options are at each step and how likely each option is to meet your goals. If treatment goals are not clear, ask your doctor to explain them in words you understand.

The Goals of the Patient

In addition to the traditional goals of tumor response, increased survival, and symptom control, older cancer patients often have goals related to quality of life. These may include maintaining physical and intellectual independence, spending quality time with family, taking trips, staying out of the hospital, or even sustaining economic stability. At times, palliative care or hospice may meet these goals better than active anticancer treatment. In addition to the medical team, older patients often turn to family, friends, and clergy for help and guidance.

5. DETERMINE IF YOU ARE FIT OR FRAIL

Deciding how to treat cancer in someone who is older requires a thorough understanding of her general health and social situation. Decisions about cancer treatment should never focus on age alone.

Age Is Not a Number

Your actual age (chronological age) has limited influence on your prognosis or on how your cancer will respond to therapy. Physiological and other changes associated with aging are more reliable in estimating an individual's vigor, life expectancy, or the risk of treatment complications. These changes include malnutrition, loss of muscle mass and strength, depression, dementia, falls, social isolation, and the ability to accomplish daily activities such as dressing, bathing, eating, shopping, housekeeping, and managing one's finances or medication.

Chronic Illnesses

Older cancer patients are likely to have chronic illnesses (comorbidity) that affect their life expectancy; the more that you have, the greater the effect. This effect has very little impact on the behavior of the cancer itself, but studies do show that comorbidity has a major impact on treatment outcome and its side effects.

6. BALANCE BENEFITS AND HARM

Studies show that physically and mentally fit older breast cancer patients respond to treatment like their younger counterparts. However, a word of caution is in order. Until recently, few studies included older individuals, and it may not be appropriate to apply these findings to the diverse group of older cancer patients.

The side effects of cancer treatment are never less in the elderly. In addition to the standard side effects, there are significant age-related toxicities to consider. Though most of these are more a function of frailty than chronological age, even the fittest senior cannot avoid the physical effects of aging. In addition to the changes in fat and muscle you see in the mirror, there are age-related changes in your kidney, liver, and digestive (gastrointestinal) functions. These changes affect how your body absorbs and metabolizes anticancer drugs and other medicines. The average older woman takes many different medicines (to control, for example, high blood pressure, high cholesterol, osteoporosis, diabetes, arthritis, etc.). This "polypharmacy" can cause undesirable side effects as many drugs interact with each other as well as the anticancer medications.

7. GET INVOLVED

Healthcare providers and family members often underestimate the physical and mental abilities of older people and their willingness to face chronic and life-threatening conditions. Studies clearly show that older patients want detailed and easily understood information about potential treatments and alternatives. Patients and families may consider cancer untreatable in the aged and may not understand the possibilities offered by treatment.

While patients with dementia pose a unique challenge, they are frequently capable of participating in goal setting and simple discussions about treatment side effects and logistics. Caring family members and friends are often able to share the patient's life story so that healthcare workers can work with them to make decisions consistent with the patient's values and desires. This communication is no substitute for a well thought out and properly executed living will or healthcare proxy.

While it is hard to face the possibility of life-threatening events at any age, it is always better to be prepared and to "put your affairs in order." In addition to estate planning and wills, it is critical that you outline your wishes regarding medical care at the end of life, and make legal provisions for someone to make those decisions if you are unable to make them for yourself.

TREATING BREAST CANCER

YOU NEED A TEAM

Cancer care changes rapidly. It is hard for a generalist to keep up to date, so referral to a specialist is essential. The needs of an older cancer patient often extend beyond the doctor's office and the traditional services provided by visiting nurses. These needs may include transportation, nutrition, emotional, financial, physical, or spiritual support. When an older woman with breast cancer is the primary caregiver for a frail or ill spouse, grandchildren, or other family members, special attention is necessary to provide for their needs as well. Older cancer patients cared for in geriatric oncology programs benefit from multidisciplinary teams of oncologists, geriatricians, psychiatrists, pharmacists, physiatrists, social workers, nurses, clergy, and dietitians, all working together as a team to identify and manage the stresses that can limit effective cancer treatment.

SURGERY

Breast surgery is a relatively low-risk operation. It is the standard of care for all women with early stage breast cancer, regardless of age. Like other treatment options, breast surgery in some older women may involve risks related to decreases in body organ function (especially heart and lung). It is essential that the surgeon and anesthetist work closely with your primary care physician (or a consultant) to fully assess and treat these problems before, during, and after the operation.

Body image is just as important to older women as to younger women. Breast-conserving surgery (lumpectomy or partial mastectomy) with postoperative radiation therapy is the procedure of choice for patients of all ages with early breast cancer. Some older women, with limited mobility or difficulties with transportation, may prefer mastectomy over the frequent visits to the hospital required for post-lumpectomy radiation therapy.

Although some have suggested that axillary lymph node dissection serves no therapeutic role in older women, the benefit of this procedure is probably no different from that experienced by younger women. Lymphedema (arm swelling after axillary lymph node dissection) can be particularly debilitating in older women with arthritis and mobility problems. Sentinel node biopsy techniques virtually eliminate this risk and should be used in all elderly women for staging and treatment decisions, even if the tumor is small.

RADIATION THERAPY

Regardless of age, radiation therapy following breast-conserving surgery significantly reduces both the risk of 5-year recurrence and 15-year breast cancer mortality. Healthy older women usually tolerate radiation therapy quite well, and even frail patients may find the side effects acceptable.

Though studies in older women have found no significant increase in side effects from radiation therapy, the fatigue that often accompanies radiation therapy can be quite profound in the elderly (even in those who are fit). Often the logistical details, like daily travel to the hospital for a 6-week course of treatment, are difficult for older people. It is important that you discuss these potential problems with your family and social worker prior to starting radiation therapy. Women who have cardiac pacemakers may need to have them moved to a location outside of the radiation therapy fields to avoid pacemaker malfunctions during treatment.

Not every elderly woman may need adjuvant radiation therapy to prevent recurrence of cancer. The Cancer and Leukemia Group B (CALGB) is currently following a group of women, 70 years and older, who have low-risk, estrogen receptor positive, node-negative tumors that are less than 2.0 cm in size. Half of the women in this group were treated with post-lumpectomy Nolvadex and radiation therapy, and the other half received Nolvadex without radiation therapy. After 8 years, the women who received radiation therapy were 5% less likely to have breast cancer recur in their breast. Though this difference was significant, it was still quite low. Since there was no difference in survival between the two groups, the CALGB suggested that breast irradiation might not be necessary in this group of low-risk older women.

Since it often takes more than 8 years for breast cancer to recur, it may be too early to use this study to make decisions about adjuvant radiation therapy. One should also keep in mind the complications that Nolvadex can cause, especially blood clots and pulmonary emboli. It does, however, seem reasonable to consider the option of doing without adjuvant radiation in women 70 years or older who have low-risk tumors (estrogen receptor positive, lymph node-negative, less than 2.0 cm in size), especially if they have serious risks factors for mastectomy or radiation therapy and no contraindication to taking Nolvadex for 5 years. The role of the aromatase inhibitors in this setting has yet to be determined, but it seems reasonable to believe that their benefit may be similar to that of Nolvadex.

Radiation therapy is particularly effective in treating bone pain caused by breast cancer metastases to the bone. A short course of radiation therapy often allows patients with advanced cancer to lower, or even eliminate, their dose of narcotic pain relievers. Although these medicines do an excellent job of controlling pain, they often cause confusion, falls, and constipation in older patients. Thus, even hospice patients suffering from localized metastatic bone pain should consider the option of palliative radiation therapy.

HORMONAL THERAPY

Since most older women have estrogen or progesterone receptor positive breast cancer, hormonal therapy is often an excellent treatment option. Aromatase inhibitors (such as Arimidex) work better and generally have fewer side effects than Nolvadex in postmenopausal women with both early stage and advanced breast cancer. However, these agents do have a tendency to make bone loss worse and increase the risk of fracture, which is of special concern for older women who have osteopenia or osteoporosis. Such a patient can still use an aromatase inhibitor if her doctor follows her bone health carefully and manages it aggressively.

Early Stage Breast Cancer: Adjuvant Hormonal Therapy

Five years of adjuvant hormonal therapy decreases breast cancer recurrence and mortality, regardless of age.

Aromatase inhibitors are 3%–5% more effective, and generally less toxic, than Nolvadex in postmenopausal women.

Since aromatase inhibitors can cause bone loss, all older women should have a bone density study (DEXA scan) before starting an aromatase inhibitor. You also should take appropriate calcium and vitamin D supplements. If you have been taking these supplements regularly and your bone density scan shows significant osteopenia or osteoporosis, you should start taking oral bisphosphonates, such as Fosamax (alendronate sodium), Actonel (risedronate sodium), or Boniva (ibandronate sodium). If you have osteopenia, but not osteoporosis, and have not been taking calcium and vitamin D, it is reasonable to try these supplements first. By following your bone density on repeated DEXA scans, your doctor can see if these oral therapies are working. Most insurance companies will pay for only one DEXA scan a year; this is usually adequate in this situation.

If these measures do not prevent bone loss, intravenous bisphosphonates such as Zometa (zoledronic acid) may allow you to remain on an aromatase inhibitor. On the other hand, if you have no major risk factors like blood clots, your doctor may consider switching to Nolvadex. It is still an excellent drug for both early stage and advanced breast cancer, and it has less risk of aggravating osteoporosis. Women who are prone to falling, or have already had a broken bone due to osteoporosis, should probably simply avoid the aromatase inhibitors altogether.

Hormonal Therapy Instead of Surgery

Hormonal therapy has an important role in treating older patients who are expected to live only a few months, who do not want surgery, or for whom surgery is too risky due to serious comorbid conditions or frailty. Such patients also are poor candidates for chemotherapy. Hormonal therapy can effectively control, and even shrink, the local breast cancer and any associated cancer in the axillary lymph nodes. It is usually tolerated quite well. Of course, the use of this "primary hormonal therapy" requires that the tumor express hormone receptors. Aromatase inhibitors are more effective and less toxic in most older women, but Nolvadex remains a viable alternative when they are contraindicated. Primary hormonal therapy is no substitute for surgery. It is much less effective than surgery at controlling the cancer.

Metastatic Breast Cancer

Metastatic breast cancer is treatable but not curable. Just as in younger patients, the goal of treatment in older patients with metastatic breast cancer is to maintain quality of life, minimize symptoms from disease, and prolong survival without causing excessive side effects. Older women are more likely than younger women to be diagnosed at a more advanced stage of breast cancer, due to a lack of screening or delays in management.

Hormone treatment should be the treatment of choice for women with estrogen receptor positive or progesterone receptor positive tumors without life-threatening disease. As with younger patients, chemotherapy is generally reserved for those whose breast cancer progresses despite hormonal therapy, or when the metastases extensively involve vital organs.

CHEMOTHERAPY

Non-frail older cancer patients respond to chemotherapy similarly to their younger counterparts. Though the side effects of cancer treatment are never less burdensome in the elderly, they can be managed by oncologists, especially geriatric oncologists, who work in teams with others who specialize in the care of the elderly. With appropriate care, healthy older women do just as well with chemotherapy as younger women.

Advances in supportive care (antinausea medicines and blood cell growth factors) have significantly decreased the side effects of chemotherapy and improved safety and the quality of life of older women with breast cancer. Nonetheless, there is risk, especially in frail patients.

Early Stage Breast Cancer: Adjuvant Chemotherapy

Recent studies show that adjuvant chemotherapy improves survival in older women with estrogen receptor negative tumors. However, older women with hormone receptor positive tumors do not benefit as much. It is important to note that women with high-grade hormone receptor positive tumors that have low levels of hormone receptors are an exception, in that they, as well as those with multiple positive axillary lymph nodes, may have some benefit to adding adjuvant chemotherapy to adjuvant hormonal therapy.

Healthy older patients can receive the same chemotherapy regimens as their younger counterparts, including those that are anthracycline-based. Older women who receive anthracycline-based regimens are at increased risk of developing congestive heart failure. The newer taxane-based regimens (such as Taxotere [docetaxel] and Cytoxan [cyclophosphamide]) may be a reasonable alternative, especially in those with a significant cardiac risk for anthracyclines. The extra toxicity caused by adding a taxane to an anthracycline-based regimen is probably justified only in those older women with aggressive high-grade breast cancers with multiple positive lymph nodes or overexpression of the HER2neu oncogene.

Approximately 25% of older women have tumors that overexpress the HER2neu oncogene, and Herceptin should be considered in their treatment regimens. It is an extremely effective adjuvant agent when given in conjunction with chemotherapy (any benefit without chemotherapy has yet to be established). It should be considered for all older patients with HER2neu positive breast cancer who do not have significant heart disease. Ongoing and careful cardiac monitoring is essential in all older patients.

Studies have shown that doctors often under treat older women with early stage breast cancers. Though the desire to minimize side effects is understandable, these doctors are not doing you any favors. Adjuvant chemotherapy is significantly less effective when it is given in lower than standard doses or when treatment is delayed. Since the goal of adjuvant chemotherapy is cure, every effort should be taken to avoid delay and dose reductions.

Metastatic Breast Cancer

Older women whose breast cancers have progressed despite hormonal therapy, or who are hormone receptor negative, have the same benefit from chemotherapy as their younger counterparts. You should not be excluded from receiving chemotherapy for advanced breast cancer. Preference should be given to chemotherapeutic drugs with safer profiles, such as weekly taxane regimens, Xeloda (capecitabine), Gemzar (gemcitabine), and Navelbine (vinorelbine). Single agent therapy is less toxic and just as effective as combination chemotherapy.

Although targeted treatments are quite effective in older patients with metastatic breast cancer, they are not without risk. Congestive heart failure due to Herceptin is probably more related to pre-existing heart problems than to age itself. There is little information available about the risks and benefits of Avastin in older patients with breast cancer, but there does appear to be an increased risk of blood clots and other vascular problems when Avastin is given in combination with chemotherapy.

COMMON TREATMENT COMPLICATIONS IN THE ELDERLY

Anemia (low red blood cell count) is common in the elderly, especially the frail elderly. It decreases the effectiveness of chemotherapy and often causes fatigue, falls, cognitive decline (for example, dementia, disorientation, or confusion), and heart problems. Therefore, it is essential that anemia be recognized and corrected with red blood cell transfusions or the appropriate use of erythropoiesis-stimulating agents like Procrit or Aranesp.

Myelosuppression (low white blood cell count) is also common in older patients getting chemotherapy or radiation therapy. Older patients with myelosuppression develop life-threatening infections more often than younger patients, and they may need to be treated in the hospital for many days. The liberal use of granulopoietic growth factors (or G-CSF, including Neupogen [filgrastim] and Neulasta [pegfilgrastim]) decreases the risk of infection and makes it possible for older women to receive full doses of potentially curative adjuvant chemotherapy.

Mucositis (mouth sores) and diarrhea can cause severe dehydration in older patients, who often are already dehydrated due to inadequate fluid intake and diuretics ("water pills" for high blood pressure or heart failure). Careful monitoring and the liberal use of antidiarrheal agents (Imodium) as well as oral and intravenous fluids are essential components in managing older cancer patients, especially those receiving 5-fluorouracil (5-FU) or Xeloda.

Kidney function declines as we age. Some of the medicines that older patients take to treat both their cancer (for example, Platinol AQ [cisplatin], Paraplatin [carboplatin], Amethopterin [methotrexate], Zometa, NSAIDs) and noncancer-related problems might make this worse. The dehydration that often accompanies cancer and its treatment can put additional stress on the kidneys. Fortunately, it is often possible to minimize these effects by carefully selecting and dosing appropriate drugs, managing "polypharmacy," and preventing dehydration.

Neurotoxicity and cognitive effects (chemo-brain) can be profoundly debilitating in patients who are already cognitively impaired (demented, disoriented, confused, etc.). Elderly patients with a history of falling, hearing loss, or peripheral neuropathy (for example, nerve damage from diabetes) have decreased energy and are highly vulnerable to neurotoxic chemotherapy like the taxanes or platinum compounds. Many of the medicines used to control nausea (antiemetics) or decrease the side effects of certain chemo-therapeutic agents are also potential neurotoxins. These include Decadron (dexamethasone) for psychosis and agitation, Zantac (ranitidine) for agitation, Benadryl (diphen-hydramine), and some of the antiemetics (sedation).

Fatigue is a near universal complaint of older cancer patients. It is particularly a problem for those who are socially isolated or dependent upon others for help with activities of daily living. It is not necessarily related to depression, but can be. Depression is quite common in the elderly. In contrast to younger patients who often respond to a cancer diagnosis with anxiety, depression is the more common disorder in older cancer patients. With proper support and medical attention, many of these patients can safely receive anticancer treatment.

Heart problems increase with age, and it is no surprise that older cancer patients have an increased risk of cardiac complications (especially congestive heart failure) from an-thracyclines, Herceptin, and other potentially cardio-toxic anticancer agents. The newer anthracycline-free, adjuvant chemotherapy regimens (like Taxotere and Cytoxan) are excellent alternatives for older women with a significant cardiac risk. Unfortunately, the woman whose breast cancer overexpresses the HER2neu oncogene has no "cardiac-safe" alternative to Herceptin. Since it is such an effective drug, in both the adjuvant and metastatic setting, it is often used (safely, with careful monitoring) in all but the most high-risk group of cardiac patients.

Osteoporosis can be made worse by the aromatase inhibitors (see the discussion on pages 122–123), the mainstay of hormonal therapy in post menopausal women with breast cancer. This side effect in turn can result in fractures, falls, and progressive debility.

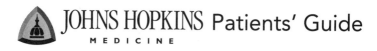

CHAPTER 11

JOHNS HOPKINS Patients' Guide

MEDICINE

Trusted Resources—Finding Additional Information About Breast Cancer and Its Treatment

For those of you wanting more information about breast cancer, there is a wealth of educational materials and resources (emotional and financial) available from a variety of credible organizations. Below is a list of trusted and useful websites and organizations that can assist you further should you choose to seek additional help.

American Cancer Society
(800) ACS-2345
http://www.cancer.org/

This national nonprofit organization provides free educational materials and offers a hotline to address questions of patients and family members dealing with all types of cancer. They can also provide support services, such as free transportation to chemotherapy treatments for patients without financial means to provide for themselves. Additionally, the national office can connect you with their local branch in your geographic region.

American Society of Plastic Surgeons

http://www.plasticsurgery.org/Patients_and_
Consumers/Procedures/Reconstructive_Procedures/
Breast_Reconstruction.html

This organization provides a helpful website that describes the various types of breast reconstruction and shows anatomic drawings of how the procedures are performed.

Breastcancer.org

http://www.breastcancer.org

Breastcancer.org is a nonprofit organization dedicated to providing the most reliable, complete, and up-to-date information about breast cancer. Their mission is to help women and their loved ones make sense of the complex medical and personal information about breast cancer, so they can make the best decisions for their lives.

Mothers Supporting Daughters with Breast Cancer

(410) 778-1982
http://www.mothersdaughters.org
Email: msdbc@verizon.net *or* lilliepie@aol.com

This is a national nonprofit organization dedicated to providing support to mothers who have daughters diagnosed with breast cancer. This organization offers a free "mother's handbook" and "daughter's companion booklet" that provide basic information about breast cancer and its treatment as well as some recommended constructive ways for mothers to provide support physically, emotionally, financially, and spiritually. The organization also "matches" mothers with mother volunteers across the country based on the daughter's (patient's) clinical picture, age at time of diagnosis, and anticipated treatment plan. They also have an online newsletter and a bulletin board for posting questions. Lillie Shockney is the "daughter" and cofounder of this organization.

National Cancer Institute (NCI)

(800) 4-CANCER (NCI's Cancer Information Service)
http://www.cancer.gov/

This organization provides information about all types of cancer, including excellent information about breast cancer, what it is, how it is treated, and where various treatment options are provided. You can request free information by calling the toll-free number.

Network of Strength (formerly known as Y-ME)

(800) 221-2141 (24-hour national hotline)
(800) 986-9505 (24-hour hotline in Spanish)
http://www.networkofstrength.org

Network of Strength is committed to providing information and support to anyone who has been touched by breast cancer. The services listed on their website include a national hotline for women needing emotional support; kid's corner; referral information for approved mammography facilities near you; public education workshops where you will find a listing of upcoming events; teen programs where you can order a video specifically for teenage girls to learn about breast cancer awareness; and a resource library that provides information about treatment modalities.

Susan G. Komen for the Cure

(877) GO-KOMEN

http://www.komen.org

This is a national volunteer organization seeking to eradicate breast cancer as a life-threatening disease, working throughout the United States and other countries to raise money for research and education, and to promote awareness. They hold more than 120 Race for the Cure events across the country as one of their primary fundraisers. The foundation is the largest private funder of breast cancer research in the United States. The Komen Alliance is a comprehensive program for the research, education, diagnosis, and treatment of breast disease. You will find information on their website about their mission, their accomplishments to date, how you can participate, grants they have funded, a national calendar of events, and other information. Komen is very big on education about the disease and on ensuring treatment for the underserved.

Young Survival Coalition

(877) YSC-1011

http://www.youngsurvival.org

Email: info@youngsurvival.org

The Young Survival Coalition (YSC) is the only international, nonprofit network of breast cancer survivors and supporters dedicated to the concerns and issues that are unique to young women and breast cancer. Through action, advocacy, and awareness, the YSC seeks to educate the medical, research, breast cancer, and legislative communities and to persuade them to address breast cancer in women 40 years of age and under. The YSC also serves as a point of contact for young women living with breast cancer.

WHERE CAN I GET HELP WITH FINANCIAL OR LEGAL CONCERNS?

Accompanying any serious illness are questions and concerns related to expenses incurred as a result of treatment, health insurance questions that can be overwhelming to try to understand or resolve alone, and sometimes even legal questions related to employment or financial matters. The following is a list of national resources to aid you in addressing these concerns.

CancerCare, Inc.

(212) 712-8400
(800) 813-HOPE
http://www.cancercare.org
Email: info@cancercare.org

CancerCare is a national nonprofit organization that provides free, professional assistance to people with any type of cancer and to their families. This organization offers education, one-on-one counseling, financial assistance for nonmedical expenses, and referrals to community services.

National Coalition for Cancer Survivorship

(301) 650-9127

(877) NCSS-YES (to order the Cancer Survival
Toolbox)

http://www.canceradvocacy.org

Email: info@canceradvocacy.org

This network of independent groups and individuals provides information and resources about cancer support,
advocacy, and quality-of-life issues and also helps cancer
patients deal with insurance issues, job discrimination issues, or other related legal matters.

Patient Advocate Foundation

(800) 532-5274

http://www.patientadvocate.org

Email: help@patientadvocate.org

This organization provides educational information about
managed care/insurance issues and legal counseling on
debt intervention, job discrimination issues, and insurance
denials of coverage.

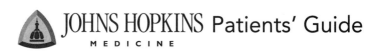

JOHNS HOPKINS Patients' Guide
MEDICINE

INFORMATION ABOUT
JOHNS HOPKINS

The Johns Hopkins Avon Foundation Breast Center

(443) 287-2778: Appointment line
(410) 614-2853: Author's direct line
Author's email: shockli@jhmi.edu
http://www.hopkinsbreastcenter.org

This breast center offers comprehensive, state-of-the-art breast cancer diagnosis and treatment. A special online feature is *Artemis*, Johns Hopkins' electronic breast cancer medical journal that you can subscribe to for free at http://www.hopkinsbreastcenter.org/artemis. It is published online monthly and provides the most up-to-date information about the latest available research results and information related to diagnosis and treatment of this disease. The website also has sections about diagnosis and treatment information, breast imaging, pathology and breast reconstruction, a breast cancer patient bill of rights, and other valuable resource information.

About Johns Hopkins Medicine

Johns Hopkins Medicine unites physicians and scientists of the Johns Hopkins University School of Medicine with the organizations, health professionals, and facilities of the Johns Hopkins Health System. Its mission is to improve the health of the community and the world by setting the standard of excellence in medical education, research, and clinical care. Diverse and inclusive, Johns Hopkins Medicine has provided international leadership in the education of physicians and medical scientists in biomedical research and in the application of medical knowledge to sustain health since The Johns Hopkins Hospital opened in 1889.

If you plan to be evaluated or treated at Johns Hopkins, you will probably meet Lillie Shockney. She interacts with patients daily and matches the team of breast cancer survivor volunteers with newly-diagnosed women based on their age, stage of disease, and anticipated treatment plan. The survivor volunteer, who has already completed the same treatment plan the patient is about to embark on, remains connected with the patient as long as the patient desires, which usually is through and beyond the end of treatment.

Check out http://www.hopkinsbreastcenter.org and click on "Upcoming Events" to see if Lillie will be in your area speaking soon.

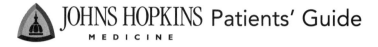
JOHNS HOPKINS Patients' Guide
MEDICINE

FURTHER READING

100 Questions and Answers About Advanced and Metastatic Breast Cancer, Lillie Shockney & Gary R. Shapiro, Jones and Bartlett Publishers, 2009.

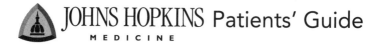

JOHNS HOPKINS Patients' Guide
M E D I C I N E

GLOSSARY

Adjuvant therapy: Treatment given after the primary treatment to increase the chances of a cure, and treatment to prevent the cancer from recurring.

Antiemetics: Antinausea medications.

Areola: The dark area around the nipple.

Aromatase inhibitors: Drugs that suppress the body's production of estrogen by reducing production of the enzyme aromatase.

Axillary lymph node dissection: Removal of the lymph nodes in the armpit during the initial surgery; the nodes are then examined by a pathologist to determine if cancerous cells are present.

Bilateral: Both sides.

Biopsy: A procedure in which cells are collected for microscopic examination.

Bone scan: An X-ray that looks for signs of metastasis.

Brachytherapy: A form of internal radiation therapy.

Breast mass: An abnormal collection of tissue within the breast.

Cancer: The presence of malignant cells.

Carcinogen: Cancer-causing substance.

Carcinomas: Cancers that form in the surface cells of different tissues.

Cells: Basic elements of tissues; the appearance and composition of individual cells are unique to the tissue they compose.

Chemo brain: Difficulty with cognitive functioning as a side effect of receiving chemotherapy.

Chemotherapy: The use of chemical agents (drugs) to systemically treat cancer.

Clinical trial: A study of a drug or treatment with a large group of people testing the treatment.

Comorbidity: A disease or disorder someone already has prior to a new diagnosis. Examples include diabetes, heart disease, and a previous history of blood clots.

Complementary therapy: Medicines used in conjunction with standard therapies.

Deep inferior epigastric perforator (DIEP) flap reconstruction: Skin and fat is transferred from the abdomen to the mastectomy site and shaped like a breast with no muscle taken.

Drains: A small tube inserted into a wound cavity to collect fluid.

Ductal carcinoma: Cancer beginning in the lining of the ducts.

Ductal carcinoma in situ (DCIS): A noninvasive cancer in which abnormal cells are found only in the lining of the milk ducts of the breast.

Ducts: The passages within the breast that bring milk from the lobules to the nipple.

Estrogen: Female hormone related to child bearing.

Estrogen receptor positive cancer: Cancer that grows more rapidly with exposure to the hormone estrogen.

Field: The treatment site.

Healthcare proxy: A document that permits a designated person to make decisions regarding your medical treatment when you are unable to do so.

HER2neu overexpression: A genetic feature of some cancers in which a receptor for human epidermal growth factor receptor 2 (HER2neu) protein, which encourages cell growth, occurs excessively due to an alteration in the HER2neu gene.

Hormonal therapy: Treatment that blocks the effects of hormones upon cancers that depend on hormones to grow (also referred to as endocrine therapy).

Hormone replacement therapy: Administration of artificial estrogen and progesterone to alleviate the symptoms of menopause and to prevent health problems experienced by postmenopausal women, particularly osteoporosis.

Incidence: The number of times a disease occurs within a population of people.

Inflammatory breast cancer: A rare but aggressive type of breast cancer characterized by symptoms resembling a skin infection or rash.

Invasive cancer: Cancer that breaks through normal breast tissue barriers and invades surrounding areas.

Latissimus dorsi reconstruction: A procedure in which the latissimus dorsi muscle (muscle on the back, below the shoulder) is used in creating a new breast following mastectomy.

Living will: A document that outlines what care you want in the event you become unable to communicate due to coma or heavy sedation.

Lobular carcinoma: Cancer formed in the lobules.

Lobular carcinoma in situ: A condition in which abnormal cells are found in the lining of the milk lobule.

Lobules: Individual glands within the lobes that secrete milk.

Lumpectomy: A medical procedure in which only the tumor and a small section of normal breast tissue are removed from the breast, leaving the breast virtually intact.

Lymph: Fluid carried through the body by the lymphatic system, composed primarily of white blood cells and diluted plasma.

Lymph nodes: Tissues in the lymphatic system that filter lymph fluid and help the immune system fight disease.

Lymphatic system: A collection of vessels with the principal functions of transporting digested fat from the intestine to the bloodstream, removing and destroying toxins from tissues, and resisting the spread of disease throughout the body.

Lymphedema: A condition in which lymph fluid collects in tissues following removal of or damage to lymph nodes during surgery, causing the limb or area of the body affected to swell.

Malignant: Cancerous; growing rapidly and out of control.

Mammogram/mammography: An X-ray examination of the breast.

Menopause: End of menstrual periods.

Metastasis, metastasize: The spread of cancer to other organ sites.

Modified radical mastectomy: A procedure in which the surgeon removes the breast, some lymph nodes under the arm, and the lining over the chest muscles.

Mortality: The statistical calculation of death rates due to a specific disease within a population.

Mutated: Altered.

Neutropenia: A condition of an abnormally low number of a particular type of white blood cell called a neutrophil. White blood cells (leukocytes) are cells in the blood that play an important role in fighting off infection.

Noninvasive cancer: Cancer confined to its tissue point of origin and not found in surrounding tissue.

Oncologist: A cancer specialist who helps determine treatment choices.

Palliative care: Care to relieve the symptoms of cancer and to keep the best quality of life for as long as possible without seeking to cure cancer.

Partial mastectomy: A procedure in which the surgeon removes the tumor, some of the normal breast tissue around it, and the lining over the chest muscles below the tumor.

Pathologist: A specialist trained to distinguish normal from abnormal cells.

Phases: A series of steps followed in clinical trials.

Placebos: An inert treatment (such as sugar pills) given in clinical trials to determine how much of a medicine's value is psychological.

Plastic surgeon: A surgical specialist who will perform any reconstruction procedures that might be required.

Post traumatic stress disorder: Emotional disorder resulting in a high level of anxiety and sometimes depression caused by a traumatic event in the past.

Primary care doctor: Regular physician who gives medical check-ups.

Progesterone: A female hormone.

Progesterone receptor positive cancer: Cancer that grows more rapidly with exposure to the hormone progesterone.

Prognosis: An estimation of the likely outcome of an illness based upon the patient's current status and the available treatments.

Protocol: The research plan for how a drug is given and to whom it is given.

Radiation oncologist: A cancer specialist who determines the amount of radiation therapy required.

Radiation therapy: Use of high-energy X-rays to kill cancer cells and shrink tumors.

Radical mastectomy (also called Halsted radical mastectomy): Removal of both of the two chest muscles, as well as the breast and lymph nodes.

Radiologist: A physician specializing in the treatment of disease using radiation therapy.

Red blood cells: Cells in the blood whose primary function is to carry oxygen to tissues.

Risk factors: Any factors that contribute to an increased possibility of getting cancer.

Selective estrogen receptor modulators (SERMs): Drugs that bind to the estrogen receptor, blocking estrogen from binding to tumor cells.

Sentinel node biopsy: Addition of dye during breast surgery to help locate the first lymph node attached to the cancerous zone; the node is then removed to prevent the spread of cancer and biopsied to determine whether cancerous cells are present.

Stage: A numerical determination of how far the cancer has progressed.

Surgical oncologist: A specialist trained in surgical removal of cancerous tumors.

Systemic treatment: A treatment that affects the whole body (the patient's whole system).

Targeted therapy: Treatment that targets specific molecules involved in carcinogenesis or tumor growth.

Transverse rectus abdominus muscle (TRAM) flap: A procedure in which a muscle from the abdomen, along with skin and fat, is transferred to the mastectomy site and shaped like a breast.

Tumor: Mass or lump of extra tissue.

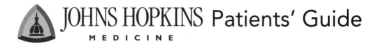

INDEX

778294

DEC 0 0 2009

DATE DUE

APR 1 9 2010	
AUG 2 5 2010	
OCT 2 0 2010	
NOV 0 3 2010	

GAYLORD   PRINTED IN U.S.A.